The CHAPTER <800> ANSWER BOOK

PATRICIA C. KIENLE

Director, Accreditation and Medication Safety
Cardinal Health Innovative Delivery Solutions

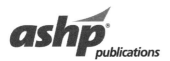

...to the publisher, ASHP, 4500 East-West Highway,

The information presented herein reflects the opinions of the contributors and advisors. It should not be interpreted as an official policy of ASHP or as an endorsement of any product.

Because of ongoing research and improvements in technology, the information and its applications contained in this text are constantly evolving and are subject to the professional judgment and interpretation of the practitioner due to the uniqueness of a clinical situation. The editors and ASHP have made reasonable efforts to ensure the accuracy and appropriateness of the information presented in this document. However, any user of this information is advised that the editors and ASHP are not responsible for the continued currency of the information, for any errors or omissions, and/or for any consequences arising from the use of the information in the document in any and all practice settings. Any reader of this document is cautioned that ASHP makes no representation, guarantee, or warranty, express or implied, as to the accuracy and appropriateness of the information contained in this document and specifically disclaims any liability to any party for the accuracy and/or completeness of the material or for any damages arising out of the use or non-use of any of the information contained in this document.

Editorial Project Manager: Ruth Bloom

Production Director: Johnna Hershey

Cover & Page Design: David Wade

Library of Congress Cataloging-in-Publication Data

Names: Kienle, Patricia C., author. | American Society of Health-System
   Pharmacists, issuing body.
Title: The chapter <800> answer book / Patricia C. Kienle.
Other titles: Guide to (work): United States pharmacopeia.
Description: Bethesda, MD : American Society of Health-System Pharmacists,
   [2017] | "Provides explanation of elements of USP Hazardous Drugs'
   Handling in Healthcare Settings and best practices to comply with the
   requirements and recommendations of the USP General Chapter"--Pref. |
   Includes bibliographical references and index.
Identifiers: LCCN 2016048833 | ISBN 9781585285730 (alk. paper)
Subjects: | MESH: Drug-Related Side Effects and Adverse Reactions--prevention
   & control | Hazardous Substances--standards | Occupational
   Exposure--prevention & control | Drug Compounding--standards
Classification: LCC RM302.5 | NLM WA 487.5.H4 | DDC 615.7/042--dc23
LC record available at https://lccn.loc.gov/2016048833

© 2017, American Society of Health-System Pharmacists, Inc. All rights reserved.

No part of this publication may be reproduced or transmitted in any form or by any means, electronic or mechanical, including photocopying, microfilming, and recording, or by any information storage and retrieval system, without written permission from the American Society of Health-System Pharmacists.

ASHP is a service mark of the American Society of Health-System Pharmacists, Inc.; registered in the U.S. Patent and Trademark Office.

ISBN: 978-1-58528-573-0

10 9 8 7 6 5 4 3 2 1

Table of Contents

Preface v
Introduction vii
Acknowledgments/Reviewers ix
Acronyms xi
List of Questions xiii

1. USP <800> Availability 1
2. General Principles of USP <800> 3
3. Contents of Sections of USP <800> 7
4. Scope of USP <800> 11
   4.1 Why is <800> Necessary? 11
   4.2 Handling Hazardous Drugs 13
   4.3 Regulations 14
   4.4 Personnel 14
   4.5 Facilities 15
5. Planning 17
   5.1 Types of Exposure 17
   5.2 NIOSH List of Hazardous Drugs 18
6. Assessment of Risk 23
7. Human Resources 29
   7.1 Medical Surveillance 29
   7.2 Designated Person 30
   7.3 Responsibilities of Compounding Personnel Training 31
   7.4 Documenting Competence 31
   7.5 Hazard Communication Plan 33
8. Personal Protective Equipment 35
   8.1 General Information 35
   8.2 Gloves 42
   8.3 Gowns 44
   8.4 Hair Covers 47
   8.5 Shoe Covers 47
   8.6 Eye Protection 48
   8.7 Respiratory Protection 49
9. Receiving Personnel: Hazardous Drug Precautions 53
10. Storage of Hazardous Drugs 59
11. Counting and Packaging Hazardous Drugs 69
12. Types of Engineering Controls 71
    12.1 General Information 71
    12.2 Containment Primary Engineering Controls for Nonsterile Compounding 73
    12.3 Containment Primary Engineering Controls for Sterile Compounding 76
13. Closed System Drug-Transfer Devices 83

14. Design of Compounding Facilities 85
    14.1 General Information 85
    14.2 Certification of Primary and Secondary Engineering Controls 93
    14.3 Anterooms 94
    14.4 Pre-Sterilization Areas for Weighing Powders 94
    14.5 Containment Secondary Engineering Controls 95
    14.6 Containment Segregated Compounding Areas 98
    14.7 Pass-Through Chambers 101
    14.8 Refrigerator and Freezer Placement 102
    14.9 Elimination of Low Volume Exemption from 2008 USP <797> 103
    14.10 Other Attributes for Designing a HD Compounding Area 104
15. Compounding Hazardous Drugs 107
16. Beyond-Use Dates 121
17. Packaging 123
18. Dispensing Hazardous Drugs 127
    18.1 Dispensing Finished Dosage Forms to Patient Care Units 127
    18.2 Dispensing Finished Dosage Forms to Ambulatory Patients 128
19. Transporting Hazardous Drugs 129
20. Administering Hazardous Drugs 131
21. Decontamination and Cleaning 135
22. Environmental Monitoring 139
23. Hazardous Waste 143
24. Spills 145
25. What Do I Do Now? 147

Future Editions 149
References 150
Appendix: Compounding Hazardous Drugs 151
Index 167

Preface

The Chapter <800> Answer Book provides an explanation of elements of USP <800> *Hazardous Drugs—Handling in Healthcare Settings* and best practices to comply with the requirements and recommendations of the USP General Chapter.

The author is a member of the USP Compounding Expert Committee, but this publication is not endorsed by or affiliated with USP.

Comments in this book are related to USP <795> and <797> from *USP 39–NF 34, 2016*. Revisions to those documents must be considered when designing policies and practices.

Patricia C. Kienle

Introduction

USP <800> *Hazardous Drugs—Handling in Healthcare Settings*[1] was published in the First Supplement to *USP 39–NF 34* on February 1, 2016, with an extended official date of July 1, 2018. One erratum was published on April 15, 2016.[2] Pharmacies and other entities where handling hazardous drugs (HDs) occur should obtain a copy of the full document. It is available from the United States Pharmacopeial Convention (USP), either as a part of the full *USP–NF* or as part of the *USP Compounding Compendium*.

The USP is recognized in the Federal Food, Drug, and Cosmetic Act as an official compendium.[3] Numbering of the chapters is significant: USP chapters numbered under <1000> are considered enforceable, and those numbered above <1000> are advisory or informational. Note that some regulatory agencies also consider those chapters above <1000> as requirements. USP uses the term *must* or *shall* when citing a requirement, but the term *should* is used when citing a recommendation.

USP is a standard-setting organization, not a regulatory or enforcement agency. Regulatory bodies (e.g., the Centers for Medicare & Medicaid Services [CMS], state boards of pharmacy, state departments of health) and accreditation organizations enforce USP standards and/or include them in their standards.

<800> is one of a number of compounding-related chapters in the *USP–NF*. It supplements but does not replace <795> *Pharmaceutical Compounding—Nonsterile Preparations* and <797> *Pharmaceutical Compounding—Sterile Preparations*. Other related USP chapters are listed in the texts of <795>, <797>, and <800>.

References

1. United States Pharmacopeial Convention. General chapter <800> hazardous drugs—handling in healthcare settings. *USP 39–NF 34 First Supplement*; 2016.
2. United States Pharmacopeial Convention. <800> Hazardous drugs—handling in healthcare settings, errata. http://www.usp.org/usp-nf/notices/hazardous-drugs-handling-healthcare-settings.
3. United States Code, Title 21, §321, http://uscode.house.gov/view.xhtml?req=%28official+compendium%29+AND+%28%28title%3A%2821%29%29%29&f=treesort&fq=true&num=0&hl=true&edition=prelim&granuleId=USC-prelim-title21-section321. Accessed September 25, 2016.

Acknowledgments

Members of the USP Expert Panel on Hazardous Drugs devoted countless volunteer hours to discussion and development of practices that make patients and healthcare personnel safer. Many thanks to Thomas Connor, Melissa McDiarmid, Eric Kastango, Kenneth Mead, Martha Polovich, Luci Power, and James Wagner and to USP staff Emily Ann Meyer, Richard Schnatz, and Jeanne Sun.

Reviewers

Lindsey B. Amerine, PharmD, MS, BCPS
Assistant Director of Pharmacy
University of North Carolina Medical Center
Associate Professor of Clinical Education
UNC Eshelman School of Pharmacy
Chapel Hill, North Carolina

Ryan A. Forrey, PharmD, MS, FASHP
Director, Pharmacy Services
Emory University Hospital Midtown
Atlanta, Georgia

Katherine Palmer, PharmD
Sterile Products Area Manager
Cedars-Sinai Pharmacy Services
Los Angeles, California

Acronyms

ACPH	air changes per hour
ADC	automated dispensing cabinet
API	active pharmaceutical ingredient
ASHP	American Society of Health-System Pharmacists
ASHRE	American Society of Heating, Refrigerating, and Air-Conditioning Engineers
ASTM	American Society for Testing and Materials
BSC	biological safety cabinet
C-PEC	containment primary engineering control
C-SCA	containment segregated compounding area
C-SEC	containment secondary engineering control
CACI	compounding aseptic containment isolator
CDC	Centers for Disease Control and Prevention
CETA	Controlled Environment Testing Association
CMS	Centers for Medicare & Medicaid Services
CSP	compounded sterile preparation
CSTD	closed system drug-transfer device
CVE	containment ventilated enclosure
EPA	Environmental Protection Agency
FDA	U.S. Food and Drug Administration
HD	hazardous drug
HEPA	high-efficiency particulate air
HVAC	heating/ventilating/air conditioning
IPA	isopropyl alcohol
ISO	International Standards Organization
IV	intravenous
IVIG	intravenous immunoglobulin
LAFW	laminar airflow workbench
MAB	monoclonal antibody
NF	National Formulary
NIOSH	National Institute for Occupational Safety and Health
ONS	Oncology Nursing Society
OSHA	Occupational Safety and Health Administration

Acronyms (continued)

PAPR	powered air-purifying respirator
PEC	primary engineering control
PPE	personal protective equipment
SDS	safety data sheet (formerly called material safety data sheet [MSDS])
sIPA	sterile 70% isopropyl alcohol
TJC	The Joint Commission
UPS	uninterrupted power source
USP	United States Pharmacopeia
wc	water column

List of Questions

Chapter 1: USP <800> Availability

1.1 Where can I find the full text of USP <800>?
1.2 When will USP <800> become official?
1.3 I have heard there may be changes to <800> that will impact remodels. How can I find out quickly?

Chapter 2: General Principles of USP <800>

2.1 Where did the information in <800> come from?
2.2 Why is the term *entity* used? Why not just call it a pharmacy?
2.3 What is the source for the list of HDs?
2.4 Do we need to include drugs on the EPA hazard list that aren't on the NIOSH list?
2.5 Can we add agents that aren't on the NIOSH list to our own facility list?
2.6 Are beta-lactam antibiotics addressed in <800>?
2.7 When must I comply with <800>?
2.8 Is there a distinction between *must* and *should* in the text of <800>?
2.9 What are the major differences between <800> and the 2008 version of USP <795> and <797>?
2.10 What containment strategies are included in <800>?
2.11 Not all HDs are antineoplastics. How much volume is needed to invest in a negative pressure room? We compound a very low volume of HDs (1-2 items a week). Does this require a whole negative room?
2.12 What are the area/facility requirements for nonsterile compounding of HDs? It sounds like USP <800> will require hoods for nonsterile compounding activities, but what if I'm just cutting tablets in half or packaging bulk tablets into unit doses?

Chapter 3: Contents of Sections of USP <800>

No questions

Chapter 4: Scope of USP <800>

4.1 Why is <800> Necessary?
4.1-1 Who has to comply with <800>?
4.1-2 What type of compounding does <800> cover?
4.1-3 Does <800> replace <797>?
4.1-4 Does <800> replace <795>?
4.1-5 Do community or mail-order pharmacies have to comply with <800>? How about a private physician's office?
4.1-6 Is a nursing station where HDs may be stored considered an "entity"?
4.1-7 Does a nursing home have to comply with <800>?
4.1-8 Who doesn't have to comply with <800>?
4.1-9 Will USP chapters be enforced at pharmaceutical wholesalers?
4.1-10 Is there any valid science behind <800>? Where can I find more information?
4.1-11 We have never had anyone injured by handling chemo agents in our facility. Why is <800> needed?
4.1-12 I've heard <800> referred to as a guideline and a standard. Which is correct? What's the difference?
4.1-13 I have heard reference to a letter that The Joint Commission sent to hospital administrators concerning risks of HDs. Where can I get a copy of the letter?

List of Questions (continued)

4.2 Handling Hazardous Drugs
- **4.2-1** What is included in *handling*?
- **4.2-2** What does *manipulation of a dosage form* mean?
- **4.2-3** Does manipulation include manual repackaging from a bottle to a unit-dose package?
- **4.2-4** Does <800> apply in emergency situations?
- **4.2-5** What is meant by the "life cycle of a HD"?
- **4.2-6** The wording about HDs isn't the same in Chapters <795>, <797>, and <800>. Which do I have to follow?

4.3 Regulations
- **4.3-1** Is <800> a regulation?
- **4.3-2** Can I select certain sections of <800> to be compliant with?
- **4.3-3** When will <800> go into effect?
- **4.3-4** Who will enforce <800> for compliance outside of pharmacy settings?
- **4.3-5** What is the difference between HDs and hazardous waste?

4.4 Personnel
- **4.4-1** Does <800> apply to the nurses in physician practices?
- **4.4-2** Our nurses mix chemo. Are they subject to <800> requirements?
- **4.4-3** Do environmental services personnel need to know about <800>?
- **4.4-4** Do pharmacy delivery drivers need to know about <800>?

4.5 Facilities
- **4.5-1** Why does <800> use the term *entity* to describe a pharmacy?
- **4.5-2** Does our outpatient pharmacy need to comply with <800>?
- **4.5-3** How does <800> apply to a patient's home?
- **4.5-4** Do wholesalers have to follow <800>?

Chapter 5: Planning

5.1 Types of Exposure
- **5.1-1** How are healthcare personnel exposed to HDs?
- **5.1-2** What are the types of exposures addressed by USP <800>?
- **5.1-3** What are the best ways to protect against exposure to HDs?
- **5.1-4** What types of HDs need to be considered—nonsterile, sterile, chemo, or others?
- **5.1-5** Are final dosage forms safer than powders?
- **5.1-6** Why are manufacturers allowed to send us products that are contaminated?

5.2 NIOSH List of Hazardous Drugs
- **5.2-1** Where can I find a list of HDs?
- **5.2-2** Can I make my own list instead of using the NIOSH list?
- **5.2-3** Why is the NIOSH list used in <800>?
- **5.2-4** What is the definition of a HD?
- **5.2-5** What are the types of HDs?
- **5.2-6** What if I don't agree with the NIOSH list? Can I eliminate some of the listed drugs from consideration at my organization?
- **5.2-7** When developing our hospital's list of HDs, do we have to include all meds on the NIOSH list?
- **5.2-8** Why are drugs other than chemo agents included on the NIOSH list?
- **5.2-9** Since <800> was approved when the 2014 NIOSH list was available, will the 2014 list be the only one that's used for <800>?

List of Questions (continued)

5.2-10 How often will the NIOSH list be updated?
5.2-11 How can I identify the HDs used in my organization?
5.2-12 How do I know if a drug that is new to the market is hazardous?
5.2-13 Why is the NIOSH list different from the list of hazardous medications we have from our waste hauler?
5.2-14 What is an *API*?
5.2-15 If I withdraw a med from a vial, is that an API because it isn't a finished dosage form until I mix it?
5.2-16 Based on NIOSH, should we change the labeling on drugs to hazardous/antineoplastic, hazardous/non-antineoplastic, and hazardous/reproductive?
5.2-17 Are all monoclonal antibodies (MABs) HDs?
5.2-18 MABs, with the exception of conjugated monoclonals, have been removed from the NIOSH list. How do you recommend monoclonals that have known teratogenic properties (i.e., rituximab, bevacizumab, cetuximab) be handled? Do these need to be prepared in a negative pressure environment? What about handling MABs for nursing?
5.2-19 Why do I need to handle megestrol as an antineoplastic? The only hazard information I see in the package insert is that it can cause malignant tumors in beagles taken for 7 years. How do you extrapolate this to a nurse pouring a liquid for a patient a few times each year who likely will not be touching it at all?
5.2-20 NIOSH lists drugs like finasteride and clonazepam in the same category. But I don't consider them the same risk. How would I know that handling should be different?
5.2-21 What about topical drugs such as diclofenac gel? It's not on the NIOSH list but definitely has the potential to affect the baby of a pregnant woman who handles it.
5.2-22 How are investigational drugs handled with respect to <800>? How should we classify investigational drugs, especially those in early clinical trials with limited safety data? It's often unclear from available information if they should be considered hazardous.
5.2-23 What are the options for investigational drug services that store HDs where sponsors require certain storage conditions? For instance, drugs must be stored in a limited access area within the investigational drug pharmacy.

Chapter 6: Assessment of Risk

6.1 What are my options to handle HDs?
6.2 What is a practical way to approach identifying the HDs I use that might be candidates for an Assessment of Risk?
6.3 Do I have to include all medications on the NIOSH list?
6.4 Our hospital decided not to include phosphenytoin and warfarin on our HD list. Is this OK?
6.5 What needs to be included in the Assessment of Risk?
6.6 Can I do an Assessment of Risk for an entire class of drugs (e.g., hormones) instead of each individual drug?
6.7 Is there a template I can use to list each drug and dosage form to determine if it's acceptable to be included in our Assessment of Risk?
6.8 Can non-antineoplastics and reproductive hazards be handled differently than antineoplastics?
6.9 Should all MABs be treated as hazardous?
6.10 Why is an Assessment of Risk allowed by <800> if all the drugs on the NIOSH list are hazardous?
6.11 When a HD is a final dosage form (e.g., tablet, capsule) and an Assessment of Risk has been performed, can this HD fall outside of the USP <800> regulation?

List of Questions (continued)

6.12 What antineoplastics don't have to be handled as HDs?
6.13 What about excluding "counting final dosage forms" when large quantity counting is performed?
6.14 How often do I need to review the Assessment of Risk?
6.15 Who needs to know that I did an Assessment of Risk?
6.16 What are some examples of alternative containment strategies?
6.17 Would the containment strategies be applied to drugs (e.g., megestrol oral suspension) if the patient receives less than the full size of the unit dose?
6.18 The NIOSH 2016 list of HDs says nurses must use double gloves for administration of anything on the HD list (even non-chemotherapy) except intact tablets or capsules. This seems excessive. Is this where the Assessment of Risk could be applied?
6.19 If I have to package methotrexate tablets, isn't the risk different for the tech who packages it versus the nurse who administers it?
6.20 Do I have to exclude packaging and counting in my Assessment of Risk?
6.21 What if I handle a non-antineoplastic HD but don't include it on my Assessment of Risk?
6.22 Can I do an Assessment of Risk for an entire class of drugs instead of listing each individual drug?

Chapter 7: Human Resources

7.1 Medical Surveillance
7.1-1 What does *medical surveillance* mean?
7.1-2 What department determines how this will work?
7.1-3 What types of medical surveillance will be required?
7.1-4 Should all employees have to sign lists acknowledging risk/NIOSH drug list?
7.1-5 Should pregnant or breast-feeding pharmacy technicians and pharmacists, or any employees trying to conceive, be removed from work duties of preparing chemo?
7.1-6 Should nurses who are pregnant or wish to become pregnant avoid taking care of patients who are on HDs due to administration and drug elimination in bodily fluids?

7.2 Designated Person
7.2-1 Who is the *designated person* mentioned in <800>?
7.2-2 Can the *designated person* be a committee instead of an individual?
7.2-3 Does the *designated person* need to be a pharmacist?
7.2-4 Does the *designated person* need to be a manager?
7.2-5 Is the *designated person* responsible for compliance with USP <800>?
7.2-6 Does oversight of handling HDs have to be the *designated person's* sole job responsibility?
7.2-7 Can the *designated person* be responsible for more than one site?
7.2-8 Where can the *designated person* obtain the necessary training for this job?
7.2-9 How much training does the *designated person* need to have?

7.3 Responsibilities of Compounding Personnel Training
7.3-1 What training is required to handle HDs?

7.4 Documenting Competence
7.4-1 What competence information has to be documented?
7.4-2 How often should training occur?
7.4-3 If we add a new drug similar to one we use, does that require full annual-type documentation?
7.4-4 Who needs to be trained on the hazards of HDs?
7.4-5 Do I still need to do the personnel training listed in <795>?
7.4-6 Do I still need to do the personnel training listed in <797>?

List of Questions (continued)

- **7.4-7** Does <800> require training separate from what we do for the hospital?
- **7.4-8** Do I need to teach my night nursing supervisors how to use the chemo hood?

7.5 Hazard Communication Plan

- **7.5-1** What is a Hazard Communication Plan?
- **7.5-2** Whose responsibility is it to develop a Hazard Communication Plan?
- **7.5-3** Is a hazardous chemical the same thing as a HD?
- **7.5-4** Do all HDs require a Safety Data Sheet (SDS)?
- **7.5-5** What are the occupational exposure limits for HDs?
- **7.5-6** Do employees have to document that they know they are working with HDs?
- **7.5-7** Do both male and female employees need to document their acknowledgment of HDs?
- **7.5-8** Where can I get an example of an employee consent form regarding exposure to HDs?

Chapter 8: Personal Protective Equipment

8.1 General Information

- **8.1-1** What does <800> require for PPE?
- **8.1-2** What are the benefits of PPE?
- **8.1-3** Are all the components of PPE needed for every activity when handling HDs?
- **8.1-4** What does *donning* and *doffing* mean?
- **8.1-5** What does *hand hygiene* mean?
- **8.1-6** When gloves are mentioned in <800>, does that mean *chemo gloves*?
- **8.1-7** What PPE needs to be worn by receiving personnel?
- **8.1-8** What PPE needs to be worn by personnel who are transporting HDs?
- **8.1-9** What PPE needs to be worn by personnel who are packaging HDs?
- **8.1-10** What PPE needs to be worn by personnel who are compounding HDs?
- **8.1-11** Does the pharmacist checking the preparation compounded in the C-PEC need to wear all PPE if he or she is not touching anything, but just looking?
- **8.1-12** If a pharmacist completes the checking of a CSP in the anteroom, does he or she need to garb?
- **8.1-13** Is additional PPE required for personnel who are compounding from powders?
- **8.1-14** My CACI technical manual states that head/hair/shoe covers are not required when compounding. Does USP supersede that?
- **8.1-15** Should PPE be donned before entering the negative pressure lab?
- **8.1-16** Is it necessary for the compounding pharmacist to remove all PPE each time he or she steps out to answer the phone?
- **8.1-17** The compounding pharmacist does all the patient counseling when new prescriptions are picked up. Does the pharmacist have to remove all PPE each time during the day when counseling a patient?
- **8.1-18** Is an N95 respirator required when compounding HDs that could cause a respiratory risk?
- **8.1-19** How do PPE requirements differ between nonsterile and sterile compounding?
- **8.1-20** Do you have to wear PPE when transporting drugs to an infusion area?
- **8.1-21** What PPE needs to be worn by personnel who are administering HDs?
- **8.1-22** What PPE needs to be worn by personnel who are discarding HD trash?
- **8.1-23** What PPE does personnel need to wear when cleaning up a spill?
- **8.1-24** Can PPE be reused?
- **8.1-25** What is meant by "reused"? Can garb be reused if removed and then donned again when required to leave the area for just a few minutes? Or does it mean reused on a different day?
- **8.1-26** Is PPE required when using a compounding isolator?

List of Questions (continued)

8.1-27 <797> allows use of a gown throughout one shift. Does this apply when compounding HDs?
8.1-28 Does the pharmacist who is checking only items need to garb?
8.1-29 What is the proper order of donning and doffing PPE for compounding HDs in a cleanroom suite (positive pressure anteroom and negative pressure buffer room)?
8.1-30 What is the proper order of donning and doffing PPE for compounding HDs in a C-SCA?
8.1-31 What is the proper order of donning and doffing PPE for compounding HDs in a compounding room for nonsterile HD preparation?

8.2 Gloves

8.2-1 Do chemo gloves have to meet a particular standard?
8.2-2 How do I know if a glove is chemo-rated?
8.2-3 Is it OK for chemo gloves to be tested per ASTM D6978 and lab chemical tested per ASTM F739?
8.2-4 Do I have to wear chemo gloves when handling non-antineoplastic HDs?
8.2-5 Do sterile chemo gloves exist?
8.2-6 When must you use sterile gloves?
8.2-7 How do I sterilize chemo gloves?
8.2-8 Is double-gloving required?
8.2-9 Why do I need to wear two pairs of gloves?
8.2-10 How can you put on two pairs of gloves? They don't fit over each other.
8.2-11 Can the inner glove be a regular glove and the outer glove be a chemo glove?
8.2-12 Are chemo gloves required when working in a compounding isolator?
8.2-13 Do I need two pairs of chemo gloves if I'm working inside a CACI?
8.2-14 We use a CACI. Is the isolator glove considered to be the second pair of gloves, or do we need two pairs plus the isolator glove?
8.2-15 Do both pairs of chemo gloves need to be sterile?
8.2-16 Do both pairs of gloves need to be made of the same material?
8.2-17 How often do gloves need to be changed?
8.2-18 Where do I find the manufacturer's information about the glove permeability?
8.2-19 How do I find a glove that I can use with carmustine or thiotepa?

8.3 Gowns

8.3-1 Do chemo gowns have to meet a particular standard?
8.3-2 How do I know if a gown is chemo-rated?
8.3-3 What documentation exists concerning permeability of chemo gowns?
8.3-4 How do I know that a particular gown will resist permeability to HDs?
8.3-5 What is the difference between gowns we use for non-HDs and those used for chemo?
8.3-6 What are chemo gowns supposed to be made of?
8.3-7 How should chemo gowns be constructed?
8.3-8 In pharmacy, we have blue plastic gowns for mixing chemo. Our nurses wear yellow isolation gowns when they administer chemo. Is this OK?
8.3-9 Can I hang my gown in the anteroom for use later in the day?
8.3-10 <797> allows a gown to be removed, retained, and used throughout the work shift if it isn't soiled. Is this allowed by <800>?
8.3-11 Can gowns be re-worn during the day if a compounder must leave the HD compounding area? How should it be removed, stored, and re-donned?
8.3-12 Are washable gowns allowed?

List of Questions (continued)

8.3-13	If we use a reusable gown service and their cleaning procedures are sufficient, does that qualify as disposable?
8.3-14	How often do gowns need to be changed?
8.3-15	How long can I use a chemo gown—one compound, one batch, or all day?
8.3-16	Why do I have to change my gown every 2-3 hours?
8.3-17	Do I need to wear a regular gown under my chemo gown?
8.3-18	Do two gowns always need to be worn when compounding or is one chemo gown OK?
8.4	**Hair Covers**
8.4-1	What is the difference between head and beard covers used for chemo and those used for non-HDs?
8.4-2	If personnel wear a head cover for religious or other reasons, is an additional hair cover necessary?
8.5	**Shoe Covers**
8.5-1	What is the difference between shoe covers used for chemo and those used for non-HDs?
8.5-2	Can I use dedicated cleanroom shoes instead of shoe covers?
8.5-3	Why does <800> require two pairs of shoe covers?
8.5-4	Do nurses need to wear shoe covers when administering chemo?
8.6	**Eye Protection**
8.6-1	What does *eye protection* mean?
8.6-2	Do I need goggles if I wear glasses?
8.6-3	When is eye protection needed?
8.6-4	I wear prescription eyeglasses. Does this qualify as eye protection?
8.6-5	I wear a face shield when I mix chemo. Is this proper eye protection?
8.6-6	Do I need eye protection when I'm mixing chemo?
8.6-7	Do I need eye protection when I'm cleaning the area inside a BSC or CACI?
8.6-8	Do I need eye protection when I'm cleaning HD areas outside a C-PEC?
8.6-9	Do I need eye protection when I'm cleaning up a spill?
8.7	**Respiratory Protection**
8.7-1	What does *respiratory protection* mean?
8.7-2	What does an N95 respirator protect against?
8.7-3	Are there respirators that are better protection than N95?
8.7-4	When is respiratory protection needed?
8.7-5	Do I need respiratory protection when I'm working in a BSC or CACI?
8.7-6	Do surgical masks provide adequate respiratory protection?
8.7-7	Since the BSC and CACI provide respiratory protection, do I need to wear a regular mask for any HD compounding?
8.7-8	Do receiving personnel need to wear respiratory protection when unpacking HDs?
8.7-9	Do I have to wear a surgical mask when compounding?
8.7-10	Do I need to wear a respirator when I'm mixing chemo?
8.7-11	Can a surgical N95 respirator be used in place of a regular N95 respirator?
8.7-12	Does everyone who works with HDs need to be fit-tested for a N95 respirator?
8.7-13	My employer has never offered fit-testing of respirators. Can pharmacy staff fit-test each other?
8.7-14	Where can I find information about fit-testing of respirators?
8.7-15	Does each person handling HDs need his or her own N95 respirator?
8.7-16	Do I need respiratory protection when I'm cleaning up a spill?

List of Questions (continued)

Chapter 9: Receiving Personnel: Hazardous Drug Precautions

9.1   What training is required for receiving personnel?
9.2   Why is delivery and acceptance of HDs covered under <800>?
9.3   Where do I open the HDs I receive from suppliers?
9.4   How do I know if a container includes a HD?
9.5   Are suppliers required to label HD containers?
9.6   Do I need a designated room for unpacking? Does it have to be negative?
9.7   Should I unpack the wholesaler tote in the chemo room?
9.8   Won't I contaminate my C-SEC if I take the wrapped HDs into it?
9.9   Could we use a powder hood to open the packages?
9.10   What regulations do manufacturers have to control the hazardous residue on the outside of their products?
9.11   Do HD totes have to be delivered to the chemo room?
9.12   Would the individual taking the plastic-wrapped package into the buffer room have to be garbed?
9.13   How should the packages of HDs be taken into the chemo room?
9.14   Is there a requirement for pressure monitoring in the receiving area to demonstrate neutral or negative air?
9.15   How should I handle receipt of antineoplastics that will be dispensed without manipulation (e.g., unit-of-use methotrexate tablets)?
9.16   What PPE should be available to receiving personnel?
9.17   Do I need to wash my hands after I remove the chemo gloves I wear when receiving and stocking chemo agents?
9.18   How should damaged or broken HD containers be handled?
9.19   What happens if a damaged package needs to be opened?
9.20   We segregate antineoplastic deliveries from our wholesaler by using a unique PO number. Do non-antineoplastics (e.g., warfarin, estrogen, fluconazole) need to be in separate totes?
9.21   Will wholesalers designate hazardous items in their ordering system?
9.22   Do I have to receive HDs in a negative pressure area?
9.23   How can I identify HD containers when they come in from suppliers?
9.24   How should HDs be packaged by suppliers?
9.25   Where should HD shipments be received?
9.26   What garb needs to be worn by receiving personnel?
9.27   What is the ideal process for receiving HDs?
9.28   Should receiving personnel open up all the boxes of chemotherapy?
9.29   What should be done when broken or damaged HDs are received?

Chapter 10: Storage of Hazardous Drugs

10.1   What are the minimum storage requirements for the location of HD storage?
10.2   Am I required to store all HDs in a negative pressure room?
10.3   Where does <800> say that I have to keep two sets of inventory—one for nonsterile and one for sterile?
10.4   Are manufacturers required to clean the outer packaging of unit-dose/unit-of-use containers?
10.5   Why do HDs need to be stored in a negative room?
10.6   Can I store HDs in the negative pressure buffer room?
10.7   Can HD and non-HD APIs be stored in the same negative pressure room if they are separated?
10.8   Do all my non-chemo agents need to be in a negative room?

List of Questions (continued)

10.9   If I use an injection for nonsterile compounding, where do I store it?
10.10 What does *antineoplastic requiring only counting or packaging* mean?
10.11 Do I have to post a sign at the front door of the pharmacy stating that HDs are stored inside?
10.12 Do oral HDs have to be stored in a negative pressure room?
10.13 What examples of alternative containment strategies could we consider for oral antineoplastic agents to allow them to be stored with regular stock?
10.14 Can I store chemo with other stock?
10.15 Can hazardous and chemotherapy drugs be stored in the same area?
10.16 Can I store all my drugs (i.e., hazardous and non-hazardous) in a single negative pressure room?
10.17 Can I store nonsterile chemo drugs in my sterile chemo room?
10.18 I don't have room in my negative pressure buffer room to store stock. Can I use a vented flammable cabinet?
10.19 I have a negative pressure room with a negative pressure cabinet that is used to store all of our HD APIs. We keep other items in that cabinet that are not hazardous. Do we need to remove the non-HD items from there?
10.20 Where can I obtain a list of hazardous medications that release volatile vapors during storage?
10.21 Does USP <797> allow storage in the buffer area?
10.22 Where do I store HDs that require refrigeration?
10.23 What are my options for storing refrigerated HDs?
10.24 Does the refrigerator have to be a negative pressure refrigerator?
10.25 I have only one pharmacy refrigerator. Can I designate one shelf to store antineoplastics?
10.26 Can I store chemo vials in smooth-coated cardboard boxes in my negative pressure buffer room?
10.27 Can I store saline vials and other similar non-hazardous items in the negative pressure buffer room?
10.28 Would it be reasonable to store a limited number of oncology support (e.g., anti-emetics) medication to be stored alongside HD in a C-SCA where the compounding takes place? It sounds like this is prohibited.
10.29 Can I use a flammable cabinet to store my chemo?
10.30 Can HDs be stored in a negative pressure cabinet located in a neutral area?
10.31 Do I understand correctly that not only do chemo agents need to be compounded in a negative pressure room, but they also need to be stored there prior to use even if they are in a manufacturer's sealed box?
10.32 Would the separation of HDs and non-HDs include storage of large quantities in original packaging prior to unpacking for prescription packaging?
10.33 What are the recommendations regarding refrigerator placement for refrigerated antineoplastic HDs? USP <797> allows placement in a negative pressure buffer room; however, <800> recommendations indicate exhaust placement near the compressor and behind unit.
10.34 Can hazardous and chemotherapy drugs be stored in the same area?
10.35 Is it acceptable to store HDs in automated dispensing cabinets?
10.36 Is it acceptable to store HDs in carousels?
10.37 If the material is not volatile, why must negative pressure storage be used?
10.38 What are the storage area requirements for a nursing unit?
10.39 Can intact (unopened) HDs be stored in neutral/normal pressure areas in addition to negative pressure rooms?
10.40 We were compliant with <797> storage; it said "separate." Why does this now need to be negative?
10.41 How do you transport inventory that has been received into a negative pressure room?
10.42 Can I use a pneumatic tube to transport chemo items to our satellite pharmacy?

List of Questions (continued)

10.43 The only injectable antineoplastic we stock is methotrexate for ectopic pregnancy. How should this be stored?
10.44 <797> states that drugs are not to be stored in the buffer area or anteroom, so why does <800> allow for storage of drugs and refrigerators in the buffer room?
10.45 Does storage in a negative pressure room include both oral and injectable medications?
10.46 My workplace is a community pharmacy. Do I need a separate room for all HDs or just for the antineoplastics?
10.47 Does the area where I place HDs awaiting return to suppliers have to be separate from the regular HD storage area?

Chapter 11: Counting and Packaging Hazardous Drugs

11.1 Can I continue to package non-antineoplastics and reproductive hazards using automated packaging machines?
11.2 How should I package unit-dose solid oral antineoplastics?
11.3 If I buy only manufacturer unit-dose or unit-of-use packages, can I store the HDs—even antineoplastics—with my regular stock?
11.4 What would be an example of how a pharmacy could package unit-dose oral antineoplastic agents and be compliant with USP <800>?
11.5 What would be an example of how a community pharmacy should count out oral antineoplastic agents?

Chapter 12: Types of Engineering Controls

12.1 General Information
12.1-1 What are the types of engineering controls?
12.1-2 How do the PECs in <800> differ from those in <797>?
12.1-3 How do the SECs in <800> differ from those in <797>?
12.1-4 How do the supplemental engineering controls in <800> differ from those in <797>?
12.1-5 What is a *C-PEC*?
12.1-6 Do certain drugs require use of a CACI instead of a BSC?
12.1-7 What are the basic requirements for a BSC for sterile compounding?
12.1-8 What is a *containment ventilated enclosure*?
12.1-9 What additional items should be considered if my CVE will have redundant HEPA filters instead of being vented to the outside?
12.1-10 What is a *containment secondary engineering control*?
12.1-11 What is a *containment segregated compounding area*?
12.1-12 What is a *supplemental engineering control*?
12.1-13 Do HEPA filters stop gases?

12.2 Containment Primary Engineering Controls for Nonsterile Compounding
12.2-1 What is a *primary engineering control*?
12.2-2 Does nonsterile HD compounding require a C-PEC?
12.2-3 What types of C-PECs are compliant for compounding nonsterile HDs?
12.2-4 Does the C-PEC used for nonsterile compounding need to be vented to the outside?
12.2-5 What does *redundant HEPA filters in series* mean?
12.2-6 Can redundant HEPA filters in series be used instead of external venting if volatile agents are compounded?

List of Questions (continued)

12.2-7 Does the pre-filter count as one of the HEPA filters?
12.2-8 Can the C-PEC for nonsterile compounding be vented into another room instead of to the outside?
12.2-9 What should I look for when buying a powder hood or CVE?
12.2-10 I make only two or three nonsterile chemo preparations a year. Can I use my BSC in the sterile compounding room to do this?
12.2-11 What is *occasional* nonsterile compounding? At what point do I need a separate hood?
12.2-12 How should community pharmacies that dispense a large number of the drugs on the NIOSH list handle <800>?
12.2-13 The only antineoplastic agent I stock is methotrexate tablets. I need to count out tablets, and sometimes there is powder in the container. How does <800> deal with that situation?
12.2-14 The only risk I have is to package unit-dose methotrexate tabs. I don't have a BSC. Can I turn off my regular laminar air flow positive pressure hood and package them there?
12.2-15 How should we prepare single doses of HDs when we need to make an oral liquid from a tablet or capsule?
12.2-16 We currently use a non-externally vented CACI for preparation of oral HDs (i.e., drawing up pediatric liquid oral HD, compounding extemporaneous HD liquids from tablets). Per <800>, will this still be acceptable or will it need to be externally vented?
12.2-17 Can nonsterile compounds be prepared in a negative pressure room in a BSC?
12.2-18 It is my understanding that when USP <800> goes into effect that all chemicals considered hazardous need to be stored in a separate room, which contains a positive pressure powder hood vented to the outside and for which all compounding must be performed. Is this correct?
12.2-19 Does the powder hood need to have a filtration system in addition to venting outside or does venting out suffice?
12.2-20 Is there an industry guidance for testing/certification of a powder hood?

12.3 Containment Primary Engineering Controls for Sterile Compounding

12.3-1 What is a *primary engineering control*?
12.3-2 What types of C-PECs are compliant for compounding sterile HDs?
12.3-3 Does the C-PEC used for sterile compounding need to be vented to the outside?
12.3-4 Can the C-PEC for sterile compounding be vented into another room instead of to the outside?
12.3-5 What should I look for when buying a C-PEC for sterile compounding?
12.3-6 I make only two or three sterile chemo preparations a year. Can I use my powder hood in the nonsterile compounding room to do this?
12.3-7 Are regular laminar air flow hoods acceptable for compounding with HDs under 800?
12.3-8 I use a positive pressure vertical laminar air flow hood for all CPSs. Will this still be allowed under <800>?
12.3-9 Do I need a separate BSC for non-antineoplastic HDs?
12.3-10 Can an acrylic glove box be used for preparation of HDs? It isn't negative pressure (there is no pressure differential), and it isn't vented.
12.3-11 Can I compound chemo and non-HDs in the same C-PEC?
12.3-12 My isolator manufacturer says I don't have to place my CACI in a negative pressure room. Is this compliant with <800>?
12.3-13 Can I compound non-hazardous CSPs in the anteroom?
12.3-14 Can I batch my chemo pre-meds in the anteroom of my negative pressure IV room?
12.3-15 Do isolators need to be vented to the outside if they have HEPA filters on the exhaust?
12.3-16 Can I place a regular hood in my negative pressure cleanroom to mix pre-meds?

List of Questions (continued)

12.3-17 USP <800> states that a LAFW cannot be used for compounding antineoplastic HDs. So, can a LAFW or CAI be used for compounding a non-antineoplastic HD?

12.3-18 Is it true that a CACI must now be installed in a segregated room? This was different from USP <797>, where if the CACI met certain air cleanliness requirements it could stand alone.

12.3-19 Must CACIs be located in a negative pressure room?

12.3-20 I have a CACI in a negative room, but it is not a cleanroom. Is this still OK with USP <800> requirements?

12.3-21 I have a CACI in a room that meets the requirements for a C-SCA. Can I still use the full BUDs listed in USP <797>?

12.3-22 Are BSCs obsolete? Do I need to get a CACI for my negative pressure cleanroom?

12.3-23 What does *class* of a BSC mean?

12.3-24 How are the types of Class II BSCs different?

12.3-25 I thought USP <797> required total exhaust BSCs.

12.3-26 I used to have a BSC that was a Class II, Type A2 unit. The exhaust was directly connected to the outside. Recently, my certifier told me I couldn't have this configuration and had to get either a new hood or change to what they term a *canopy* connection. Why?

12.3-27 How do I know that my BSC or CACI is working correctly?

Chapter 13: Closed System Drug-Transfer Devices

13.1 What is a *CSTD*?

13.2 Does <800> require the use of CSTDs for compounding HDs?

13.3 Do CSTDs have to be used when compounding in a CACI?

13.4 Does <800> require the use of CSTDs for administering HDs?

13.5 Do we need to use CSTDs for drugs such as chloramphenicol?

13.6 Is <800> requiring or recommending the use of CSTDs for more than just antineoplastic drugs?

13.7 Can I use a CSTD instead of a hood for occasional HD compounding?

13.8 USP <797> allows compounding an occasional HD in a BSC in a positive pressure room as long as a CSTD is used. Will this be acceptable under USP <800>?

13.9 Are CSTDs approved by the FDA?

13.10 Does the OMB code that some CSTD suppliers use mean that they are approved by the FDA?

13.11 How do I know if the CSTD we want to use actually works?

13.12 Can nursing use a different CSTD for administration than we do in the pharmacy for compounding?

13.13 <800> says "CSTDs known to be physically or chemically incompatible with a specific HD must not be used for that HD."[1] I assume a CSTD could be physically incompatible because of physical dimensions, shape, composition, etc., but how could it be chemically incompatible?

Chapter 14: Design of Compounding Facilities

14.1 General Information

14.1-1 What are the minimum facility requirements for compounding HDs?

14.1-2 What is an *ACPH*?

14.1-3 What are the significant differences between USP <797> and USP <800> regarding requirements for negative pressure rooms and hoods?

14.1-4 Is there a way to look at the current (allowed by <797>) options versus the upcoming (allowed by <800>) options for placement of chemo hoods in different types of allowable rooms?

14.1-5 What does *fixed walls* mean?

List of Questions (continued)

14.1-6   Do the walls have to go from floor to ceiling?
14.1-7   Can I use plastic curtains or drapes to define the hazardous room?
14.1-8   Can I have a room with hard walls and use a plastic drape or strips for the doorway?
14.1-9   Can modular cleanrooms be used?
14.1-10 Must *fixed walls* be totally solid? Is a soft-wall system using a solid steel frame affixed to the floor and ceiling OK?
14.1-11 How much volume is needed to invest in a negative pressure room? We compound a very low volume of HDs, maybe one or two per week.
14.1-12 I have an ISO 7 positive pressure anteroom that opens up into two separate buffer rooms: one ISO 7 positive pressure room for non-hazardous sterile compounding and one ISO 7 negative pressure room for chemo compounding. The hoods and the rooms meet <797> requirements and are certified every 6 months. Do I have to build a new negative pressure cleanroom to meet <800>?
14.1-13 How do the PECs and the SECs differ from 797?
14.1-14 Do we need a separate room to do antineoplastic compounding?
14.1-15 Do I have to mix my chemo in a C-SCA?
14.1-16 Do nonsterile, non-antineoplastic, hazardous medications need to be compounded/prepared in a negative pressure environment?
14.1-17 We are in the process of building a pharmacy compounding room for nonsterile compounding only (no sterile compounding). Is it possible to compound both non-hazardous and hazardous mixtures in one compounding room?
14.1-18 What does *negative pressure* mean?
14.1-19 What does *separate* mean?
14.1-20 Can the negative pressure be greater than 0.03" wc?
14.1-21 Is there a requirement for pressure gauges?
14.1-22 What does *vented to the outside* mean?
14.1-23 What does *external venting* mean?
14.1-24 Does the external vent need to go to the roof?
14.1-25 Why is venting to the outside of the building needed?
14.1-26 What does a *classified room* mean?
14.1-27 What is *unclassified* space?
14.1-28 What ISO classification is required for a cleanroom?
14.1-29 What ISO classification is required for a C-SCA?
14.1-30 Can HDs be mixed outside a cleanroom?
14.1-31 I have a non-ISO 7 room with a CACI, 12 ACPH, and negative pressure. Will this environment be acceptable to compound HDs under <800>?
14.1-32 Is a negative pressure room required under <800>?
14.1-33 If I handle only HD liquids or semisolids where no particles, aerosols, or gases are produced, do I still need to compound those HDs in a negative room?
14.1-34 What constitutes a *low volume exemption* from <800> requirements?
14.1-35 Why did the allowance for *low volume* chemo sites that was allowed in <797> get removed from <800>?
14.1-36 Is it acceptable to prepare HDs in a BSC or CACI in a positive pressure cleanroom?
14.1-37 Do negative pressure rooms protect the employees in the room?
14.1-38 Are ACPH calculated using supply air or exhaust air?
14.1-39 If the HDs I use are not volatile, why do I need negative pressure and external venting?
14.1-40 Does *unclassified room* mean it doesn't meet <800> requirements?

List of Questions (continued)

14.1-41 Do I need an area for compounding nonsterile HDs?
14.1-42 *Occasional* nonsterile compounding is a subjective term. How many compounds are *occasional*?
14.1-43 Where does a sink need to be placed?
14.1-44 Can the sink be outside of the C-SCA?
14.1-45 Why does a sink need to be at least 1 meter away from the hood?
14.1-46 Can I turn off my hood when I am not using it?
14.1-47 Why is there a range for negative pressure?
14.1-48 Can the HD (negative) room be accessed through the positive pressure buffer room?
14.1-49 Can I have a pass-through between the positive pressure anteroom and the negative pressure buffer room?
14.1-50 Can I have a pass-through between the general pharmacy area and the negative pressure buffer room?
14.1-51 What are the requirements and recommendations for a pass-through chamber?
14.1-52 Can I have a pass-through refrigerator into the negative pressure buffer room?
14.1-53 Can I have a cart pass-through (a roll-up door) open into the negative pressure buffer room?
14.1-54 What kind of finishes do I need to use for floors, walls, and ceilings?

14.2   Certification of Primary and Secondary Engineering Controls
14.2-1 How often does certification of the hoods and rooms need to occur?
14.2-2 What documents should my certifier reference on certification reports?

14.3   Anterooms
14.3-1 What is the requirement for an anteroom?
14.3-2 Can I make both the anteroom and buffer room negative pressure?
14.3-3 Why does the anteroom to a chemo room need to be ISO 7 and not ISO 8?
14.3-4 Do negative rooms used only for compounding nonsterile HDs (no sterile compounding) require an anteroom?
14.3-5 Does a C-SCA require an anteroom?

14.4   Pre-Sterilization Areas for Weighing Powders
14.4-1 Where should HD powders be weighed for preparation of sterile HD CSPs?
14.4-2 Can I weigh powders in a negative pressure anteroom?

14.5   Containment Secondary Engineering Controls
14.5-1 What are *C-SECs*?
14.5-2 How is a C-SEC in <800> different from a SEC for HDs as described in <797>?
14.5-3 What are the minimum requirements for a room/suite to compound HDs with the full BUDs allowed by <797>?
14.5-4 Does the exhaust air from a SEC room need to be HEPA filtered?
14.5-5 Can a negative pressure room be vented to the outside only through the BSC exhaust?
14.5-6 Can I use plastic curtains to separate the anteroom from the buffer room?
14.5-7 Does *fixed walls* mean I can't use a modular design?
14.5-8 Is a C-SCA different from a C-SEC?
14.5-9 What are the minimum requirements for a C-SCA, and what are the BUD limits?
14.5-10 Why would I choose to build a HD cleanroom instead of a C-SCA?
14.5-11 A segregated compounding area in <797> can be used only for low-risk preparations. Is that restriction also in <800>?
14.5-12 Can a negative room be too negative?
14.5-13 The door to my negative buffer room won't stay closed. Why does this happen?

List of Questions (continued)

14.5-14 I have a CACI in a room. Does the room itself need to be negative pressure, or is it enough if the CACI vents to the outside?

14.5-15 Do ceilings really need to be caulked in place under <800>?

14.5-16 Why do I need to place my CACI in a negative room if the manufacturer says I don't have to place it in ISO 7?

14.5-17 Do all HDs have to be compounded in a negative pressure room or just antineoplastic drugs?

14.5-18 Is there a statement in <800> about not compounding non-antineoplastic HDs in a negative pressure room?

14.5-19 Are there examples of designs for a C-SEC that I can use to explain the requirements?

14.5-20 Should the un-gowning area be inside the negative pressure room or outside of it?

14.5-21 Can a CVE used for non-hazardous compounding and a separate CVE used for hazardous compounding be in the same C-SCA?

14.6 Containment Segregated Compounding Area

14.6-1 What is a *C-SCA*?

14.6-2 Can the C-SCA be an *area* and not a *room*?

14.6-3 What is the difference between a negative pressure cleanroom and a C-SCA?

14.6-4 Is a C-SCA in <797> the same as a C-SCA in <800>?

14.6-5 Does a C-SCA have to be negative pressure?

14.6-6 Does a C-SCA have to contain HEPA-filtered ceiling air?

14.6-7 Does a C-SCA require an anteroom?

14.6-8 How big does the perimeter in a C-SCA need to be?

14.6-9 What is the purpose of the perimeter in a C-SCA? What can be inside of the perimeter? What needs to be outside the perimeter?

14.6-10 Is there an example of a design for a C-SCA that I can use to explain the requirements?

14.6-11 Should the un-gowning area be inside the negative pressure room or outside of it?

14.7 Pass-Through Chambers

14.7-1 What is a *pass-through chamber*?

14.7-2 Are there specific structural requirements for a pass-through?

14.7-3 How can I be sure a pass-through chamber isn't allowing particles into the chemo room?

14.7-4 Does a pass-through chamber into a chemo room need to be negative pressure?

14.7-5 Is a pass-through chamber the same as a pass-through window?

14.7-6 Is a pass-through chamber the same as what I have in my compounding isolator?

14.7-7 Is a pass-through chamber the same as a cart pass-through or a pass-through refrigerator?

14.7-8 Can I place a pass-through chamber between the main pharmacy and the chemo room?

14.7-9 Can I place a pass-through chamber between the anteroom and the chemo room?

14.7-10 Can I place a cart pass-through into the chemo room?

14.7-11 Can I place a pass-through refrigerator between the main pharmacy and the chemo room?

14.7-12 Can I place a pass-through refrigerator between the anteroom and the chemo room?

14.7-13 Can I place a pass-through refrigerator between a negative HD storage room and my negative buffer room?

14.8 Refrigerator and Freezer Placement

14.8-1 Can I put a refrigerator or freezer in my negative cleanroom or C-SCA?

14.8-2 How can we put bulk storage and refrigerators in the buffer zone? I thought <797> was against it.

14.8-3 Are we allowed to have a refrigerator in the negative pressure room to store refrigerated antineoplastics?

14.8-4 Do I have to place a refrigerator in the compounding area?

List of Questions (continued)

14.8-5 Does USP <800> mention anything about a pass-through refrigerator for chemo?

14.9 Elimination of Low Volume Exemption from 2008 USP <797>

14.9-1 I have been using the exemption in <797> for low volume of chemo preparations, so my chemo hood is in my regular buffer room. I don't see this listed in <800>. Has the requirement changed?

14.9-2 I compound only one or two chemos a week. I have only one IV room, and it's positive pressure. Why can't I continue to compound them in my IV room?

14.9-3 I cannot get approval to build a negative pressure cleanroom. What are my options?

14.10 Other Attributes for Designing a HD Compounding Area

14.10-1 What type of sink do I need, and where should it be placed?

14.10-2 Can I put shelving in my cleanroom or C-SCA?

14.10-3 Can I put a refrigerator in my cleanroom or C-SCA?

14.10-4 Can I put a printer in my cleanroom or C-SCA?

14.10-5 What type of finishes for the floors, walls, and ceilings do I need?

14.10-6 Shouldn't all surfaces for HD compounding (sterile and nonsterile) be "smooth, impervious, free from cracks and crevices, and non-shedding"? Why is this listed only under Nonsterile Compounding in USP <800>?

14.10-7 Do I need to have the BSC, CACI, or room on emergency power?

Chapter 15: Compounding Hazardous Drugs

15.1 What type of policies should I have?

15.2 In 2006, ASHP published guidelines on handling HDs including a detailed process for decontaminating the final prepared CSP. Does <800> require use of the same steps?

15.3 What are good sources to review for developing policies?

15.4 What is an *API*?

15.5 Is it OK to compound non-HDs in the negative pressure hood and room?

15.6 Do nonsterile, non-antineoplastic hazardous medications need to be compounded and prepared in a negative pressure environment?

15.7 For non-antineoplastic hazardous oral solutions, does drawing up patient-specific doses from a bulk bottle need to be done in a negative pressure room?

15.8 If I need to crush tablets to make a solution, where do I do that?

15.9 Can I compound nonsterile HDs in an open room?

15.10 Do I have to package methotrexate tablets in a CVE?

15.11 Do I have to split methotrexate tablets in a CVE?

15.12 I mix about 200 grams of a hormone cream at one time but dispense it in 30-gram containers. After I make the 200 grams, can I store it outside the negative pressure area and place 30 grams in a container when I need to?

15.13 We have a compliant BSC in a compliant cleanroom for HDs. Once or twice a year, we need to weigh out HD APIs in our BSC. Is this OK?

15.14 Will USP <800> allow an exemption for nursing to draw up methotrexate in the emergency department?

15.15 When is a HD not a HD? When I dissolve it in liquid or add it to a cream or ointment, does it become non-hazardous?

15.16 When is a compounded topical cream able to leave the negative pressure area?

15.17 Is it OK to prepare HDs in the same Class II Type B2 BSC where biological preparations occur?

15.18 What is the best way to handle bacillus Calmette-Guérin?

15.19 Why do I have to doff garb in the chemo room?

List of Questions (continued)

15.20 Can the check of chemo items occur in the anteroom, or does it need to occur in the buffer room?
15.21 Why do I have to label non-chemo meds made in a BSC with PPE precautions?
15.22 Why do I need to use a plastic-backed preparation mat for compounding HDs?
15.23 Should the plastic-backed preparation mat be replaced each time the hood is cleaned?
15.24 Does the plastic-backed mat need to be sterile when used for sterile compounding?
15.25 Is it OK to spray alcohol?
15.26 How frequently should we change the spray bottles of cleaners?
15.27 How should alcohol be applied in the C-PEC if I can't use a spray?
15.28 Is it OK to use pre-saturated gauze to disinfect vials?
15.29 Are CSTDs required in an isolator?
15.30 Can corrugated cardboard be used in a negative pressure cleanroom?
15.31 Is there a disposable mortar and pestle that can be used for compounding HDs?
15.32 Can I use alcohol gel instead of washing my hands when I take off my gloves?
15.33 Do I have to record lot numbers for every chemo?
15.34 Is a different type of technique used for compounding HDs than used for regular compounding?
15.35 Does negative pressure technique have to be used if closed CSTDs are used for compounding?
15.36 What is the recommendation for HDs that are needed emergently (e.g., valproic acid, fosphenytoin)? Should they be compounded in the pharmacy's BSC rather than in the Emergency Department or intensive care unit?
15.37 If <800> requires compounding in negative pressure rooms, why is there a need to discuss compounding outside of the proper facility?

Chapter 16: Beyond-Use Dates

16.1 Why is there no BUD information in USP <800>?
16.2 How will a 12-hour BUD work if the drug needs to run longer than that?
16.3 We have a C-SCA and prepare HD pumps for home care patients. The infusion is started within 12 hours of being compounded, but it runs for 144 hours. Is this OK?
16.4 Is the maximum BUD for nonsterile compounding described in USP <795>? I don't understand why this isn't included in USP <800>.

Chapter 17: Packaging

17.1 Is unit dosing of antineoplastics considered compounding, and does it have to be performed in a controlled environment?
17.2 Is it OK to use a packaging machine to unit dose HDs?
17.3 Which oral dosage forms of HDs don't require counting in negative rooms?
17.4 Even though <800> allows antineoplastics in final forms that require only counting or packaging, why wouldn't I use a powder hood or BSC to pre-package them?
17.5 What precautions are needed for crushing tablets or opening capsules of HDs?
17.6 Our obstetric department uses misoprostol in 25-mcg tablets. They are available only in 100-mcg tablets. How can we best comply with their needs?
17.7 Do patient-specific doses of antineoplastic oral solution HDs need to be drawn up in a negative pressure room? How about non-antineoplastic HD oral solutions?
17.8 Is it OK to use a packaging machine for HDs that aren't antineoplastic?
17.9 How are hospitals managing warfarin administration if it requires cutting/splitting of tablets?
17.10 Who crushes tablets for nasogastric tube administration—pharmacy or nursing?
17.11 What precautions should be taken when unit-dosing liquids are on the HD list?

List of Questions (continued)

17.12 If pharmacy unit doses a HD, does that mean it's a final dosage form?
17.13 After I have compounded or packaged nonsterile antineoplastic agents into the finished dosage form, how do I need to store them prior to dispensing or patient pick-up?
17.14 USP <800> says that when you make a non-HD in a chemo hood, you have to label it with PPE handling precautions. Where are the precautions listed? Are they in the Safety Data Sheet, Department of Transportation information, or somewhere else?

Chapter 18: Dispensing Hazardous Drugs

18.1 Do I need a separate counting tray for each different HD?
18.1 **Dispensing Finished Dosage Forms to Patient Care Units**
18.1-1 What precautions need to be taken for chemo bags between the pharmacy, and where will they be administered?
18.1-2 Is it OK to store HDs in ADCs?
18.1-3 Is it OK to deliver HDs in pneumatic tubes?
18.2 **Dispensing Finished Dosage Forms to Ambulatory Patients**
18.2-1 What precautions need to be taken for an oral chemo dispensed and waiting for patient pick-up?
18.2-2 Do I need to decontaminate a nonsterile HD preparation after I make it?
18.2-3 The NIOSH list states that single gloves should be worn with administration from unit-dose packages. How does this impact community pharmacies where pharmacists and technicians have the potential to touch these final dosage forms during dispensing?

Chapter 19: Transporting Hazardous Drugs

19.1 Why can't pneumatic tubes be used for transporting HDs?
19.2 Can HDs be transported in tubes, robots, patient carts, etc.?
19.3 Can volunteers transport finished chemo to our oncology center?

Chapter 20: Administering Hazardous Drugs

20.1 What PPE is required for administration of parenteral HDs?
20.2 Is PPE (other than gloves) required for the administration of oral HDs?
20.3 Is there a list of recommended PPE to wear based on the dosage form administered?
20.4 If nurses have to wear gloves for administration of HDs, do they need to change the gloves between patients?
20.5 Can a nurse crush a HD tablet at the bedside?
20.6 What does <800> mean by a *plastic pouch* to contain particles?
20.7 What PPE should a nurse wear when crushing HDs?
20.8 Our Emergency Department nurses might administer IM methotrexate at night when the pharmacy is closed. Do they need to take any precautions when they prepare the dose?
20.9 Why do nurses need to use a CSTD when administering chemo?
20.10 What precautions must be made for administering oral chemotherapy through a feeding tube? There are issues in mixing the doses administered to the patient, but there are no CSTDs for this process.
20.11 What happens when a stat oxytocin drip is needed?
20.12 What precautions must be in place for the nursing staff who administer HDs to patients in an outpatient infusion setting?
20.13 Does a non-antineoplastic drug like premixed oxytocin require a CSTD?
20.14 Where can I find nursing competencies?

List of Questions (continued)

Chapter 21: Decontamination and Cleaning

- 21.1 What is the difference between cleaning and decontamination?
- 21.2 How is cleaning a chemo hood different from what's done for the regular hood?
- 21.3 Do I need to wear PPE when cleaning?
- 21.4 Is it OK for Environmental Services to clean the floors while we are compounding?
- 21.5 What agents deactivate HDs?
- 21.6 What agents decontaminate HD areas?
- 21.7 What agents clean HD areas?
- 21.8 What agents disinfect HD areas?
- 21.9 Is alcohol sufficient to decontaminate and clean the HD areas?
- 21.10 Who should clean the BSC and CACI?
- 21.11 Who should clean the SECs?
- 21.12 Are there specific cleaning guidelines under USP <800>?
- 21.13 Is there a single process I can use to deactivate all HDs?
- 21.14 What concentration of bleach should I use?
- 21.15 How do I know I am using the correct dilutions of decontamination and cleaning solutions?
- 21.16 Do I need to clean the whole hood between mixing different chemo preps?
- 21.17 What should I use to decontaminate the chemo hood between chemo preps?
- 21.18 Why shouldn't I use a spray bottle of alcohol?
- 21.19 What should I use to disinfect the chemo hood between preparations?
- 21.20 How do I decontaminate the floor?
- 21.21 How often should I use sterile alcohol to clean the floor?
- 21.22 Are specific cleaning supplies required by USP <800>?
- 21.23 Are reusable mops acceptable to use?
- 21.24 What is the best way to monitor that cleaning has been done?
- 21.25 What do I do about a rusty hood?
- 21.26 How can I tell if we are removing the contaminants?

Chapter 22: Environmental Monitoring

- 22.1 What types of quality assurance and quality control activities are required or recommended in USP <800>?
- 22.2 USP <795> doesn't include a requirement for microbial monitoring for nonsterile compounding areas. Should this be considered?
- 22.3 Is surface sampling the only quality point that needs to be considered?
- 22.4 Are wipe samples required?
- 22.5 Are there different requirements if we are using an isolator instead of a BSC?
- 22.6 How often should wipe samples be collected?
- 22.7 Where should wipe samples be collected?
- 22.8 Are we likely to find contamination?
- 22.9 What drugs are commonly assayed?
- 22.10 How many surface samples are usually taken?
- 22.11 What action do we need to take if antineoplastic contamination is found? How can we get the level to zero?
- 22.12 What is the responsibility of the *designated person* regarding surface sampling results?
- 22.13 What are the acceptable limits for the results of HD surface contamination?
- 22.14 Once contamination is found on wipe samples and the issue is addressed, should we expect the next levels to show zero contamination?
- 22.15 Why is surface sampling only *recommended* and *not required*?

List of Questions (continued)

Chapter 23: Hazardous Waste

23.1 Does it seem like the section about disposal got the short end of the stick? It just says "all applicable federal, state, and local regulations."[1] Disposition of hazardous components within the healthcare setting seems to me to be just as important as the other areas listed in the chapter.
23.2 Is proper disposal of HDs part of a compounder's responsibilities under USP <800>?
23.3 Who can provide the information our health system needs to know about disposal of HDs and the federal and state requirements?
23.4 Does pharmacy need to control the handling of hazardous materials for the health system?

Chapter 24: Spills

24.1 What is a *spill*?
24.2 Are antineoplastic agents the only concern?
24.3 What is a *spill kit*?
24.4 What spill kit contents does USP <800> require?
24.5 Is there a standard spill kit that I can purchase?
24.6 Where do spill kits need to be located?
24.7 What should be in a spill kit?
24.8 How big a spill can a spill kit handle?
24.9 What resources can I use to develop a policy concerning spill cleanup?
24.10 Who should clean up a spill?
24.11 If a facility contracts Hazmat for all hazardous spills, do infusion staff still need to be trained in HD spill cleanup, and are spill kits required in cleanrooms?
24.12 What is the best way to test our policy and procedure?

Chapter 25: What Do I Do Now?

25.1 I'm overwhelmed with this information. Where do I start?
25.2 Where can I find a gap analysis?
25.3 What can I do to comply with <800> while waiting for capital improvements to my compounding facility to be completed?
25.4 Is there a template Action Plan I could use to start assessing the compliance at my organization?

Reference

1. United States Pharmacopeial Convention. General chapter <800> hazardous drugs—handling in healthcare settings. *USP 40–NF 35*; 2017.

USP <800> AVAILABILITY   1

1.1 Where can I find the full text of USP <800>?

USP publishes the *USP Compounding Compendium*. It contains all of the major compounding chapters: <795> *Pharmaceutical Compounding—Nonsterile Preparations,* <797> *Pharmaceutical Compounding—Sterile Preparations,* and <800>*Hazardous Drugs—Handling in Healthcare Settings* as well as all the other chapters that are referenced in those three core compounding chapters. Additionally, the *General Notices* that apply to compounding and compounding monographs are included. They are available through USP at www.usp.org as an annual subscription.

Your subscription allows you to re-download updates throughout your subscription year. Be sure to do that each February, June, and November so you have the most current versions of existing chapters and any new *General Notices, General Chapters,* or monographs that were completed in the prior months.

1.2 When will USP <800> become official?

USP <800> will be a federally enforceable standard as of July 1, 2018.

1.3 I have heard there may be changes to <800> that will impact remodels. How can I find out quickly?

<800> is final. The only changes to this initial version will be errata, which will be posted on www.usp.org. One errata notice was published in June 2016 (www.usp.org/usp-nf/official-text/errata-table?mono_num=7808) removing the requirement to high-efficiency particulate air (HEPA)-filtered air vented from the negative room. Future revisions of <800> will go through a public comment period—as all new and revised USP chapters do—so you will have notice of any future changes.

GENERAL PRINCIPLES OF USP <800>

2.1 Where did the information in <800> come from?

Information about risks to personnel from hazardous drugs (HDs) has been in the medical literature since the 1970s. ASHP's first guidance on handling HDs was published in 1985 as the *Technical Assistance Bulletin on Handling Cytotoxic Drugs in Hospitals*.[1] Revisions to that document were published in 1990[2] and 2006.[3] A new revision is anticipated in summer 2017. The National Institute for Occupational Safety and Health (NIOSH) published the *Alert* on *Preventing Occupational Exposure to Antineoplastic and Other Hazardous Drugs in Health Care Settings* in 2004.[4] The *Alert* included a list of HDs, which was updated in 2010, 2012, 2014, and 2016.[5] The ASHP and NIOSH documents form the core of the information in <800>. The Occupational Safety and Health Administration (OSHA) information on controlling occupational exposure to HDs,[6] other professional organizational guidance (e.g., from the Oncology Nursing Society), scientific publications,[7] and best practices that have evolved since these documents were published have also been incorporated into <800>.

2.2 Why is the term *entity* used? Why not just call it a pharmacy?

<800> applies to many more healthcare settings than pharmacies. Physician offices, clinics, veterinary offices, and many other locations handle HDs. When you see the term *entity* in <800>, apply it to your setting.

2.3 What is the source for the list of HDs?

The NIOSH list of antineoplastic and other HDs[5] is the hazardous drug list used in <800>.

2.4 Do we need to include drugs on the EPA hazard list that aren't on the NIOSH list?

No. The NIOSH list includes drugs that are hazardous to personnel; it's the focus of <800>. The Environmental Protection Agency (EPA) hazardous materials list includes drugs and other substances that are hazardous to the environment. That is not the focus of <800>. Some drugs appear on both lists, so compliance with both <800> (for protecting personnel) and the EPA (for protecting the environment) needs to be addressed.

2.5 Can we add agents that aren't on the NIOSH list to our own facility list?

Yes, but there is no requirement to do so.

2.6 Are beta-lactam antibiotics addressed in <800>?

No, because they are not on the NIOSH list of HDs. However, you can include agents other than those listed on the NIOSH list in your policies if you choose to.

2.7 When must I comply with <800>?

<800> is official and federally enforceable on July 1, 2018. However, states or other regulatory agencies, accreditation organizations, and entity policy may require compliance before that date. This is all about limiting occupational exposure, so the sooner compliance is achieved, the safer your workplace will be.

2.8 Is there a distinction between *must* and *should* in the text of <800>?

Yes. *Must* is used for a requirement; *should* is used for a recommendation.

2.9 What are the major differences between <800> and the 2008 version of USP <795> and <797>?

Major differences include the following:

- *Scope.* <795> and <797> deal with receipt, compounding, and storage up to the point of administration. The scope of <800> spans more activities because its intent is to protect all healthcare workers. <800> includes protection of healthcare workers from the time the HD is received, through and including administration of the HD and disposal of HD waste.

- *Elimination of the "low use" exemption.* <797> allowed placement of a biological safety cabinet (BSC) or compounding aseptic containment isolator (CACI) in a positive pressure room, provided only a low volume of HDs was compounded. This is not allowed by <800>. All HD compounding must occur in a negative pressure room.

- *Requirement to compound nonsterile HDs in a negative pressure room.* USP <795> *Pharmaceutical Compounding—Nonsterile Preparations* provides general guidance for compounding nonsterile HDs but does not specify required elements. <800> includes requirements for compounding nonsterile HDs.

- *Requirement for use of closed system drug-transfer devices (CSTDs) when administering antineoplastic agents.* The scope of <795> and <797> stops when administration of the drug begins. The scope of <800> is greater and includes requirements for worker protection through administration and disposal of the HD. CSTDs provide protection for those individuals who administer HDs and are required by <800> when the dosage form allows their use.

2.10 What containment strategies are included in <800>?

There are three major containment strategies: engineering controls, personal protective equipment, and work practices.

2.11 Not all HDs are antineoplastics. How much volume is needed to invest in a negative pressure room? We compound a very low volume of HDs (1-2 items a week). Does this require a whole negative room?

There is no "low use" exemption in <800>, and it will be removed from <797> so the two chapters are in synch. If you compound any active pharmaceutical ingredients (APIs) on the NIOSH list or any antineoplastics, you need the proper facilities. The two options in <800>

are either a negative pressure cleanroom suite (positive pressure anteroom opening into a negative pressure cleanroom) or a containment segregated compounding area (C-SCA), which needs to be negative but does not need to be an International Standards Organization (ISO) 7 cleanroom.

If you compound only those drugs that are final U.S. Food and Drug Administration (FDA)-approved dosage forms and none is antineoplastic, you may be able to establish alternative containment strategies and/or work practices through an Assessment of Risk. In that case, you might not need a negative pressure room if you can identify other practices that mitigate the risk.

2.12 What are the area/facility requirements for nonsterile compounding of HDs? It sounds like USP <800> will require hoods for nonsterile compounding activities, but what if I'm just cutting tablets in half or packaging bulk tablets into unit doses?

If you are manipulating antineoplastic agents—even oral tablets—you need to do this in the proper facility. Manipulation of HDs that aren't antineoplastic may be described in your Assessment of Risk. (See Section 6 on Assessment of Risk.) <800> permits use of the BSC or CACI in your sterile negative pressure compounding room for occasional nonsterile use, as long as the stipulations listed in <800> are followed. If you do this routinely, you need to have the proper equipment for nonsterile HD compounding/repackaging.

CONTENTS OF SECTIONS OF USP <800>

3

USP <800> *Hazardous Drugs—Handling in Healthcare Settings* is divided into sections. The key elements in each section are listed below.

Introduction and Scope
- List of personnel to whom <800> applies
- Examples of healthcare settings where <800> applies
- Types of activities described in <800>
- Organization of the Chapter

List of Hazardous Drugs
- Use of the NIOSH list of hazardous drugs
  * For which drugs all containment strategies in <800> must be used
  * For which drugs and dosage forms you may develop an Assessment of Risk, identify alternative containment strategies and/or work practices, and implement those strategies and practices
- What the Assessment of Risk must contain

Types of Exposure
- Types of activities that have a risk of exposure
- Potential opportunities for exposure

Responsibilities of Personnel Handling Hazardous Drugs
- Assignment of a person who is responsible for oversight of handling hazardous drugs in your organization
- Responsibilities of all personnel who handled hazardous drugs

Facilities and Engineering Controls
- Facility requirements for receiving hazardous drugs
- Facility requirements for storage of hazardous drugs
- Facility requirements for compounding nonsterile hazardous drugs
- Facilities requirements for compounding sterile hazardous drugs
- Primary engineering controls ("hoods")
- Secondary engineering controls (the rooms in which "hoods" are located)
- Requirements for negative pressure in rooms
- Requirements for external venting of "hoods" and rooms
- Use of closed system drug-transfer devices (CSTDs)

Environmental Quality and Control
- Wipe sampling of hazardous drug areas

Personal Protective Equipment (PPE)
- Gloves
- Gowns
- Hair covers
- Shoe covers
- Sleeve covers
- Goggles
- Face protection
- Respirators and masks
- Disposal of used PPE

Hazard Communication Program
- Occupational Safety and Health Administration (OSHA) requirements
- Safety Data Sheets
- Need for personnel to document that they understand the risks of handling hazardous drugs

Personnel Training
- Training
- Competency documentation
- Frequency of personnel competency assessment

Receiving
- Established policies and procedures
- How hazardous drugs should be packaged by suppliers
- Required PPE
- Requirement for spill kit
- How to handle damaged packages

Labeling, Packaging, Transport, and Disposal
- Labeling requirements
- Packaging requirements
- Requirements when mailing hazardous drugs
- Requirements of environmental services personnel

Dispensing Final Dosage Forms
- How to handle hazardous drug preparations waiting for patient pick-up
- How to handle hazardous drug preparations sent to patient care units
- Use of dedicated dispensing equipment
- Restriction of use of automated counting or packaging equipment

Compounding
- Need to comply with USP <795> when storing and compounding nonsterile hazardous drugs
- Need to comply with USP <797> when storing and compounding sterile hazardous drugs
- Use of plastic-backed protective pads
- Handling bulk containers of liquids and active pharmaceutical ingredients (APIs)

Administering
- Use of protective devices when administering hazardous drugs
- Required PPE when administering hazardous drugs
- Use of CSTDs
- Restriction when crushing, splitting, or opening oral dosage forms of hazardous drugs

Deactivating, Decontaminating, Cleaning, and Disinfecting
- Need for policies and procedures
- When deactivation is needed and example agents to use
- When decontamination is needed and example agents to use
- When cleaning is needed and example agents to use
- When disinfection in needed and example agents to use
- Wiping down hazardous drug containers
- Cleaning under the work tray of a biological safety cabinet (BSC) or a compounding aseptic containment isolator (CACI)

Spill Control
- Need for proper training of personnel
- Procedures to incorporate for spill cleanup

Documentation and Standard Operating Procedures
- Development of policies and procedures
- Frequency of review of policies and procedures
- List of policies and procedures
- OSHA requirements

Medical Surveillance
- Overview of a medical surveillance program
- Elements that should be included in your organization's medical surveillance program
- Information about chronic exposure
- Information about acute exposure (spills)

Glossary
- Definition of terms used in <800>

Appendix 1: Acronyms
- Explanation of acronyms used in <800>

Appendix 2: Examples of Design for Hazardous Drugs Compounding Areas
- Examples of nonsterile hazardous drug compounding rooms
- Examples of sterile hazardous drug compounding rooms
- Examples of a room used for nonsterile and sterile compounding

Appendix 3: Types of Biological Safety Cabinets
- Description of classes of BSCs
- Description of types of BSCs

References
- References used in the development of <800>

SCOPE OF USP <800> 4

4.1 WHY IS <800> NECESSARY?

4.1-1 Who has to comply with <800>?

All healthcare personnel must comply. This includes anyone who handles hazardous drugs (HDs)—personnel involved in receiving, storage, compounding, transporting, administering, disposal, or spill cleanup.

4.1-2 What type of compounding does <800> cover?

Both nonsterile and sterile compounding when HDs are handled.

4.1-3 Does <800> replace <797>?

No. <800> provides the information on handling HDs. It must be used in conjunction with <797> for sterile compounding.

4.1-4 Does <800> replace <795>?

No. <800> provides the information on handling HDs. It must be used in conjunction with <795> for nonsterile compounding.

4.1-5 Do community or mail-order pharmacies have to comply with <800>? How about a private physician's office?

All healthcare sites must comply with <800>. This includes pharmacies of any type, physician offices and clinics, veterinarian offices, and any other healthcare setting where HDs are handled.

4.1-6 Is a nursing station where HDs may be stored considered an "entity"?

Yes, since a nursing station is part of a healthcare setting.

4.1-7 Does a nursing home have to comply with <800>?

Yes, because a long-term care facility is a healthcare facility.

4.1-8 Who doesn't have to comply with <800>?

The scope of <800> is healthcare personnel. Manufacturing and supply chain personnel who handle the HDs before they get to a healthcare site are not included in <800>, although their workplaces require safety strategies from different agencies such as Occupational Safety and

Health Administration (OSHA). Patients' homes are not included in <800>, because they are not healthcare settings. However, home health workers are part of the healthcare team; their safety should be addressed with facility policies.

4.1-9 Will USP chapters be enforced at pharmaceutical wholesalers?

Manufacturers and distributors aren't considered healthcare settings, so <800> is out of scope for those facilities. However, other USP chapters may apply in those sites such as ones on Good Distribution Practices. Additionally, because suppliers respond to customer requests, they may implement changes so their customers are compliant.

4.1-10 Is there any valid science behind <800>? Where can I find more information?

The medical literature includes worker safety issues since the 1970s. <800> includes a listing of references. Other excellent sources of information are the web site maintained by National Institute for Occupational Safety and Health (NIOSH), which has a frequent update of new literature published (see: http://www.cdc.gov/niosh/topics/antineoplastic/default.html) and information on the OSHA Safety and Health Topics web page (see https://www.osha.gov/SLTC/hazardousdrugs/index.html).

4.1-11 We have never had anyone injured by handling chemo agents in our facility. Why is <800> needed?

You are fortunate if that is the case. However, most places don't know this information because it would require extensive medical surveillance to determine it. Harm often isn't identified when only small numbers of personnel are evaluated. Occupational risk is generally determined by large cohorts with controlled conditions. This situation doesn't exist at an individual site.

4.1-12 I've heard <800> referred to as a guideline and a standard. Which is correct? What's the difference?

<800> is a federally enforceable standard. Healthcare facilities that handle HDs are required to comply with <800>. It's not a guideline; you cannot select certain aspects to consider and not address other elements of it. However, using the Assessment of Risk approach, you can define alternative methods to comply with some of the requirements.

4.1-13 I have heard reference to a letter that The Joint Commission sent to hospital administrators concerning risks of HDs. Where can I get a copy of the letter?

OSHA, NIOSH, and The Joint Commission sent a letter to all hospital administrators in April 2011 concerning HD exposure and risks to healthcare personnel. It is available at https://www.osha.gov/ooc/drug-letter.pdf. Note that the NIOSH list of HDs has been updated since the letter was written.

4.2 HANDLING HAZARDOUS DRUGS

4.2-1 What is included in *handling*?

<800> is designed to protect healthcare workers from unintentional exposure to drugs that are hazardous to personnel. Most unintentional exposure comes from touching, inhaling, or ingesting these agents. <800> lists potential opportunities for exposure including receipt, transport, dispensing, compounding, mixing, manipulating dosage forms (e.g., crushing or splitting tablets or opening capsules), administering, cleaning up spills, and handling waste.

4.2-2 What does *manipulation of a dosage form* mean?

Manipulation includes, but is not limited to, counting (although there is an exception allowed for some situations); placement into prescription containers, unit-dose, or unit-of-use packaging; splitting tablets; opening capsules; compounding nonsterile forms (e.g., making a suspension from tablets); drawing up a dose; or compounding a sterile preparation.

4.2-3 Does manipulation include manual repackaging from a bottle to a unit-dose package?

It does, but <800> has a potential allowance for that activity. Antineoplastics that need to be only counted or packaged can have alternative containment or work practices defined in the organization's Assessment of Risk. Non-antineoplastics and reproductive hazards can have final dosage forms defined in the organization's Assessment of Risk. However, consider what risks might be present for counting or packaging oral antineoplastic agents. Even bottles of tablets could have broken tablets inside it.

4.2-4 Does <800> apply in emergency situations?

Yes, the requirement to protect employees from harm also applies in emergencies. From a practical perspective, evaluate the type of urgent situation. Antineoplastic stat orders still need all the containment protection and work practices defined in <800>. Stat requirements for those HDs that are not antineoplastic, such as the need to mix a fosphenytoin infusion in an Emergency Department without 24/7 pharmacy coverage, should be addressed in the entity's Assessment of Risk.

4.2-5 What is meant by the "life cycle of a HD"?

The scope of <800> starts with receipt of the drug and ends with administration and disposal. As you review where and how HDs are used in your organization, trace that entire cycle.

4.2-6 The wording about HDs isn't the same in Chapters <795>, <797>, and <800>. Which do I have to follow?

<800> is the definitive standard concerning HDs. The information in <795> does not conflict with <800>. The information in <797> will be harmonized with <800> and will refer issues of HDs to <800>.

4.3 REGULATIONS

4.3-1 Is <800> a regulation?

It is a federally enforceable standard. States and other regulatory agencies, accreditation organizations, and health-system policies may include <800> requirements.

4.3-2 Can I select certain sections of <800> to be compliant with?

No, you need to comply with the entire standard. However, there is an allowance for an Assessment of Risk for certain dosage forms of specific HDs. You are able to comply with <800> if the Assessment of Risk is completed, documented, and reviewed at least annually.

4.3-3 When will <800> go into effect?

It will be official on July 1, 2018. However, some regulatory agencies, accreditation organizations, or other policy-making entities (e.g., a health system) may expect compliance earlier than that date.

4.3-4 Who will enforce <800> for compliance outside of pharmacy settings?

The U.S. Food and Drug Administration (FDA) can. States determine how they will enforce any standards. Accreditation organizations will likely incorporate <800> in their standards.

4.3-5 What is the difference between HDs and hazardous waste?

The HDs included in <800> are those that NIOSH has identified as causing harm to personnel. Hazardous waste regulations are defined by the Environmental Protection Agency (EPA) (see www.epa.gov) and are harmful to the environment; these are not the focus of <800>. Some drugs are listed on both the NIOSH list and the EPA list.

4.4 PERSONNEL

4.4-1 Does <800> apply to the nurses in physician practices?

Yes. It applies to all healthcare workers.

4.4-2 Our nurses mix chemo. Are they subject to <800> requirements?

Yes. It applies to all healthcare workers.

4.4-3 Do environmental services personnel need to know about <800>?

Yes. It applies to all healthcare workers. Any healthcare personnel who handle HDs need to be aware of the risks. This includes environmental services personnel.

4.4-4 Do pharmacy delivery drivers need to know about <800>?

Yes. It applies to all healthcare workers. If their responsibility includes handling HDs, they must be informed of the risk of HDs.

4.5 FACILITIES

4.5-1 Why does <800> use the term *entity* to describe a pharmacy?

Entity is used to include all areas where HDs may be handled. It's not limited to a pharmacy but also includes physician offices, outpatient and community pharmacies, clinics, veterinary offices, and any other place where healthcare is provided.

4.5-2 Does our outpatient pharmacy need to comply with <800>?

Yes. All healthcare facilities need to comply with <800>. Most outpatient pharmacies have several of the drugs included on the table of antineoplastic drugs on the NIOSH list of HDs as well as a number of the drugs on the tables of non-antineoplastic agents and reproductive hazardous HDs. These can be addressed by an Assessment of Risk if the entity chooses to do it.

4.5-3 How does <800> apply to a patient's home?

It doesn't because the home is not a healthcare setting. However, it may apply to home healthcare workers who should be included in the entity's policies and procedures.

4.5-4 Do wholesalers have to follow <800>?

Manufacturers, wholesalers, and suppliers are not healthcare facilities, so <800> does not apply to them. However, most suppliers want to respond to their customer needs so they have incorporated elements of <800> where possible.

PLANNING 5

(See Sections 1, 2, and 3 in USP <800>.)

5.1 TYPES OF EXPOSURE

5.1-1 How are healthcare personnel exposed to HDs?

<800> is focused on minimizing unintentional exposure to hazardous drugs (HDs). Healthcare workers could be unintentionally exposed by touching surfaces contaminated with HD residue, inhaling the residue, or ingesting the agents. Contamination could be on the outside of packages received in the organization, on the outside of sterile or nonsterile products compounded, on work surfaces or breakroom tables, or on any number of other containers or surfaces. Pharmacy personnel who compound HDs and nurses and others who administer HDs could have the drugs splashed or spilled or even inadvertently injected by a needle stick. Environmental services personnel could be exposed to HDs when removing linens from a patient's room or removing trash from the pharmacy or patient care unit.

5.1-2 What are the types of exposures addressed by USP <800>?

Exposure can occur when hazardous drugs are inhaled, touched, injected, or ingested.

5.1-3 What are the best ways to protect against exposure to HDs?

The National Institute for Occupational Safety and Health (NIOSH) uses a framework of a Hierarchy of Controls to assess protection. (See http://www.cdc.gov/niosh/topics/hierarchy/.) *Elimination*—physically removing the hazard—and *substitution*—replacing the hazard—are effective controls, but they don't work in this situation. We need to provide these HDs for patient care.

The three remaining controls are incorporated into <800> containment strategies:
1. Engineering controls, which isolate personnel from the hazard.
2. Administrative controls, which define the way people work.
3. Personal protective equipment (PPE), which protect personnel.

5.1-4 What types of HDs need to be considered—nonsterile, sterile, chemo, or others?

All of them—check the NIOSH list of HDs[5] for all the agents that must be evaluated.

5.1-5 Are final dosage forms safer than powders?

Generally, yes, but be sure to assess what other healthcare personnel may be doing with the dosage forms dispensed. The *NIOSH Alert* notes that:

Some drugs defined as hazardous may not pose a significant risk of direct occupational exposure because of their dosage formulation (for example, coated tablets or capsules—solid, intact medications that are administered to patients without modifying the formulation). However, they may pose a risk if solid drug formulations are altered, such as by crushing tablets or making solutions from them outside a ventilated cabinet.[4]

5.1-6 Why are manufacturers allowed to send us products that are contaminated?

There is no current requirement to mandate manufacturers to ensure the outside of their vials and packaging is free from contamination. The scope of <800> doesn't extend to manufacturers or suppliers.

5.2 NIOSH LIST OF HAZARDOUS DRUGS

5.2-1 Where can I find a list of HDs?

<800> uses the NIOSH list of HDs.[5] This is the list you need to use to be compliant with <800>. The NIOSH list sorts HDs into three tables: (1) antineoplastic agents, (2) non-antineoplastic agents, and (3) reproductive hazards.

5.2-2 Can I make my own list instead of using the NIOSH list?

No, but you can add items to your organization's list that aren't on the NIOSH list.

5.2-3 Why is the NIOSH list used in <800>?

The NIOSH list is an existing list that has been scientifically vetted and reviewed by experts. It is a publically available list, which is updated as new agents enter the market. The process for updating is announced in the *Federal Register* so is open for anyone to provide comments.

5.2-4 What is the definition of a HD?

The definition of a HD was first published in the 1990 *ASHP Technical Assistance Bulletin on Handling Cytotoxic and Hazardous Drugs*.[2] With slight changes, the definition was used in the 2004 *NIOSH Alert* on *Preventing Occupational Exposure to Antineoplastic and Other Hazardous Drugs in Health Care Settings*,[4] the 2006 *ASHP Guidelines on Handling Hazardous Drugs*,[3] and in <800>.[8]

A drug is defined as hazardous if it exhibits any of the following characteristics:

- Carcinogenicity
- Teratogenicity or developmental toxicity
- Reproductive toxicity in humans
- Organ toxicity at low doses in humans or animals
- Genotoxicity

If a new drug, which has not yet been considered by NIOSH, mimics existing HDs in structure or toxicity it is also considered hazardous.

5.2-5 What are the types of HDs?

HDs can be grouped by the definition of a HD (carcinogenic, teratogenic, or a developmental toxin; reproductive toxin; organotoxin; or genotoxin). They may also be grouped into the tables that NIOSH uses: antineoplastic, non-antineoplastic, or reproductive hazards.

5.2-6 What if I don't agree with the NIOSH list? Can I eliminate some of the listed drugs from consideration at my organization?

No, you need to consider all of the drugs in all three tables of the NIOSH list. All of these drugs meet the definition of a HD. However, you can assess the dosage forms that you handle of the non-antineoplastic and reproductive HDs and include them in your Assessment of Risk.

5.2-7 When developing our hospital's list of HDs, do we have to include all meds on the NIOSH list?

You have to review the list and identify the drugs and the dosage forms you use. You probably do not handle all the drugs on the list; those you don't handle don't need to be on your list.

5.2-8 Why are drugs other than chemo agents included on the NIOSH list?

Drugs other than antineoplastics are included on the NIOSH list because they meet the definition of a HD. It's not only carcinogens that are included; there are also teratogenic or developmental toxins, reproductive toxins, organotoxins, or genotoxins.

5.2-9 Since <800> was approved when the 2014 NIOSH list was available, will the 2014 list be the only one that's used for <800>?

No, whatever NIOSH list is current is the list you must use. The 2016 list was published in September 2016.[7] When an updated NIOSH list is published, it is the list that must be used to be compliant with <800>.

5.2-10 How often will the NIOSH list be updated?

NIOSH plans to update the list about every 2 years.

5.2-11 How can I identify the HDs used in my organization?

Match the drugs and dosage forms on the NIOSH list to any use of those agents in your organization. Pharmacy purchasing records are a logical place to start but also include review of any other department that could potentially receive medications such as Materials Management, oncology clinics, and physician practices associated with your health system. If Patient Assistance Programs or Compassionate Use Programs are used at your organization, or if patients or practitioners may bring in their own medications, be sure to include them in your assessment.

5.2-12 How do I know if a drug that is new to the market is hazardous?

If it is similar to an existing HD in structure or toxicity, consider it hazardous until it is more extensively evaluated. If the manufacturer defines it as hazardous in the product labeling, it would also need to be considered hazardous.

5.2-13 Why is the NIOSH list different from the list of hazardous medications we have from our waste hauler?

The NIOSH list concerns drugs that are hazardous to personnel. The list from your waste hauler concerns drugs that are hazardous to the environment. Some drugs are on both lists.

5.2-14 What is an *API*?

USP <800> defines an *active pharmaceutical ingredient (API)* as "any substance or mixture of substances intended to be used in the compounding of a drug preparation, thereby becoming the active ingredient in that preparation and furnishing pharmacological activity or other direct effect in the diagnosis, cure, mitigation, treatment, or prevention of disease in humans and animals or affecting the structure and function of the body."[8] Powders and other raw materials are API. Final dosage forms of U.S. Food and Drug Administration (FDA)-approved medications are not API, although API was used in their creation.

5.2-15 If I withdraw a med from a vial, is that an API because it isn't a finished dosage form until I mix it?

No. The contents of an FDA-approved dosage form (e.g., a vial) are not an API; API is the raw material.

5.2-16 Based on NIOSH, should we change the labeling on drugs to hazardous/antineoplastic, hazardous/non-antineoplastic, and hazardous/reproductive?

<800> does not require you to change the way you label medications. You could choose to do that in your policies, but there is no requirement to do so.

5.2-17 Are all monoclonal antibodies (MABs) HDs?

No. Check the NIOSH list of HDs[5] for those agents that need to be included in your review.

5.2-18 MABs, with the exception of conjugated monoclonals, have been removed from the NIOSH list. How do you recommend monoclonals that have known teratogenic properties (i.e., rituximab, bevacizumab, cetuximab) be handled? Do these need to be prepared in a negative pressure environment? What about handling MABs for nursing?

Drugs that are on the NIOSH list must be evaluated; others—such as those MABs you mention—can be added if your assessment shows that they also need containment properties and/or work practices defined in <800>.

5.2-19 Why do I need to handle megestrol as an antineoplastic? The only hazard information I see in the package insert is that it can cause malignant tumors in beagles taken for 7 years. How do you extrapolate this to a nurse pouring a liquid for a patient a few times each year who likely will not be touching it at all?

Megestrol is classified as an antineoplastic agent. Antineoplastic agents that must be manipulated, such as a nurse pouring a liquid for a patient, need to be prepared under conditions that are compliant with <800>. Additionally, the Centers for Medicare & Medicaid Services (CMS) Hospital Conditions of Participation[9] and accreditation organization standards require that doses are provided in a ready-to-administer dosage form. Consider unit-dosing this in the pharmacy for patient-specific doses.

5.2-20 NIOSH lists drugs like finasteride and clonazepam in the same category. But I don't consider them the same risk. How would I know that handling should be different?

Clonazepam and finasteride are listed in the table of reproductive hazards. That doesn't mean the risks are the same. Look under the heading for Reason for Listing. Clonazepam is there because of increased risk of congenital abnormalities when taken in the first trimester. Finasteride is there because women should not handle crushed or broken finasteride tablets when they are pregnant or may potentially be pregnant due to potential risk to a male fetus. If you choose to do an Assessment of Risk (rather than handle all the drugs and dosage forms the same way), you need to take into account these situational risks when you develop your alternative strategies for containment.

5.2-21 What about topical drugs such as diclofenac gel? It's not on the NIOSH list but definitely has the potential to affect the baby of a pregnant woman who handles it.

You can include drugs and dosage forms of agents that are not on the NIOSH list on your own list. Additionally, you can contact NIOSH or watch for the *Federal Register* notice about updates to the list if you think other drugs should be added to the NIOSH list.

5.2-22 How are investigational drugs handled with respect to <800>? How should we classify investigational drugs, especially those in early clinical trials with limited safety data? It's often unclear from available information if they should be considered hazardous.

If a drug mimics an existing agent identified as hazardous either in structure or toxicity, you need to consider it hazardous until further information is known.

5.2-23 What options are available for investigational drug services that store HDs where sponsors require certain storage conditions? For instance, drugs must be stored in a limited access area within the investigational drug pharmacy.

This will depend on the structure of your facility. If it is where you have an existing negative pressure room, could you store it separately but in that room? If you need to store it in one place (e.g., within negative space in your investigational drug pharmacy) and transport it to another room to compound it, you can develop a procedure that incorporates the required storage elements and a safe method to transport it (e.g., in a container that minimizes the risk of breakage or leakage).

ASSESSMENT OF RISK 6

6.1 What are my options to handle HDs?

<800> details the containment strategies and work practices that are required. For antineoplastics (other than those that require only counting or packaging), you must use all the containment strategies and work practices listed in <800>. For antineoplastics that require only counting or packaging, non-antineoplastics, or reproductive hazardous agents, you have two options: (1) treat them with all the containment strategies and work practices listed in <800> or (2) perform an Assessment of Risk to develop and use alternative containment strategies and/or work practices.

6.2 What is a practical way to approach identifying the HDs I use that might be candidates for an Assessment of Risk?

Here's one approach:
- Print out the National Institute of Occupational Safety and Health (NIOSH) list of hazardous drugs (HDs).
- Identify the drugs and dosage forms that you handle in your organization.
- Sort them into five lists:
  1. Active pharmaceutical ingredient (API) of any drug on the NIOSH list of HDs.
  2. Antineoplastic drugs and dosage forms that must be manipulated.
  3. Antineoplastic drugs and dosage forms that require only counting or packaging.
  4. Non-antineoplastic drugs and dosage forms.
  5. Reproductive HDs and dosage forms.

API of any of the drugs on the NIOSH list of HDs must be handled with all the elements listed in <800>. Antineoplastics that must be manipulated must be handled with all the elements listed in <800>. You can then assess the agents on your other categories that might be acceptable to handle with other containment strategies or work practices. Consider the risks to personnel. For example, methotrexate tablets may require only packaging, but it would be best to do that in the negative pressure engineering controls you already have. It would be more of a risk to pharmacy personnel who are packaging it than to the nurse who is provided a ready-to-administer unit-dose package.

6.3 Do I have to include all medications on the NIOSH list?

You need to review the NIOSH list of HDs and identify the drugs and dosage forms you handle. You probably do not use all the drugs on the list; those you don't handle do not need to be on your list.

6.4 Our hospital decided not to include phosphenytoin and warfarin on our HD list. Is this OK?

No. You need to include them on your list. All of the agents listed on the NIOSH list of HDs[5] need to be included on your list. You may entity-exempt some of the agents from all of the requirements of <800>, but you must identify the alternative containment strategies and/or work practices that you use to protect employees.

6.5 What needs to be included in the Assessment of Risk?

You need to consider the type of HD (antineoplastic, non-antineoplastic, or reproductive hazard), the dosage forms of each of those drugs that you handle, the risk of exposure to personnel, the packaging of the drug, and what manipulations you have to perform to get it to a finished dosage form.

6.6 Can I do an Assessment of Risk for an entire class of drugs (e.g., hormones) instead of each individual drug?

No. <800> requires the Assessment of Risk to be specific to the drug and to a particular dosage form. You may find that certain subsets of drugs and dosage forms will use the same alternative containment strategy or work practice, but your entity's list must be specific to the drug and dosage form.

6.7 Is there a template I can use to list each drug and dosage form to determine if it's acceptable to be included in our Assessment of Risk?

<800> does not require a specific form. A spreadsheet with the drug, dosage form, and <800> requirements could be developed. See **Exhibit 6-1** for an Assessment of Risk template that could be used to assess each drug and dosage form used.

6.8 Can non-antineoplastics and reproductive hazards be handled differently than antineoplastics?

Yes, if you perform an Assessment of Risk to identify and implement alternative containment strategies and work practices.

6.9 Should all MABs be treated as hazardous?

Not all monoclonal antibodies (MABs) are on the NIOSH list of HDs. You must treat the ones that are on the list as hazardous. You also may add other agents to your list.

6.10 Why is an Assessment of Risk allowed by <800> if all the drugs on the NIOSH list are hazardous?

An Assessment of Risk is allowed because not all dosage forms may have the same level of risk. Working with powders or crushing tablets is more of a risk of exposure than handling a manufacturer's unit-dose tablet. Mixing intravenous (IV) solutions is more of a risk than purchasing pre-mixed solutions from a manufacturer or U.S. Food and Drug Administration (FDA)-registered outsourcing facility. <800> applies to all healthcare facilities where HDs are handled including health-system pharmacies, community pharmacies, physician offices, and other locations. Not all entities manipulate HDs to the same degree.

EXHIBIT 6-1 Hazardous Drug Assessment of Risk

Active pharmaceutical ingredient (API) of any hazardous drug (HD) on the NIOSH list or any antineoplastic agent that needs to be manipulated may NOT be considered for the Assessment of Risk; all containment strategies and work practices included in USP <800> must be followed.

DRUG _____DOSAGE FORM _____

Indicate status based on 2016 NIOSH List of Hazardous Drugs

	Final dosage form of antineoplastic that requires only counting or packaging
	Non-antineoplastic
	Reproductive hazard

Reason for exemption: _____

NOTE: This is a summary of requirements. Full requirements are listed in USP <795>, <797>, <800>, the *NIOSH Alert* and List of Hazardous Drugs, and health-system policy and procedure.

Activity	USP <800> Requirement and NIOSH Recommendation	Organizational Policy		
		Follow <800>	N/A	Entity Exemption
Purchasing				
Receipt	Unpack in neutral/normal pressure area. Spill kit and respirator available.			
Transport from Receipt to Storage	In container that minimizes risk of breakage or leakage			
Storage	Separate from non-HD, in separate room that is negative pressure, externally vented, and has at least 12 ACPH			
Transport from Storage to Compounding area(s)	In container that minimizes risk of breakage or leakage			
Transport from Storage to Dispensing area(s)	In container that minimizes risk of breakage or leakage			
Nonsterile Compounding area(s)	Meets USP <795> and <800> requirements			
Sterile Compounding area(s)	Meets USP <797> and <800> requirements			
Prepackaging area(s)	Meets USP <795> and <800> requirements and NIOSH HD list recommendations			
Splitting or crushing or withdrawing parenteral dose for placement into another container in patient care or procedural area	Meets USP <795> and <800> requirements and NIOSH HD list recommendations			

EXHIBIT 6-1 Hazardous Drug Assessment of Risk (continued)

Activity	USP <800> Requirement and NIOSH Recommendation	Organizational Policy		
		Follow <800>	N/A	Entity Exemption
Transport finished preparations to HD administration area(s)	In container that minimizes risk of breakage or leakage			
Transport finished preparations to holding area for patient pick-up	In container that minimizes risk of breakage or leakage			
Storage of finished preparations waiting for patient pick-up	No further containment unless required by manufacturer			
Transport finished preparations to off-site administration areas	In container that minimizes risk of breakage or leakage			
Ship finished prescription to patient or to other location	Consult transport information on Safety Data Sheets			
Deactivating, decontaminating, cleaning, and disinfecting compounding and administration areas	Deactivation/decontamination with an EPA-registered oxidizer Clean with a germicidal detergent Disinfect with alcohol			
Administration	Use of CSTDs when the dosage form allows			
Disposal	Per federal and state requirements and health-system policies			
Handling spills	Spill kit and respirator			

NOTES:

Approved by HD Committee on_____

Annual Review:

ACPH: air changes per hour; CSTD: closed system drug-transfer device; EPA: Environmental Protection Agency; NIOSH: National Institute for Occupational Safety and Health

6.11 When a HD is a final dosage form (e.g., tablet, capsule) and an Assessment of Risk has been performed, can this HD fall outside of the USP <800> regulation?

It is still a HD, so it is within the requirements of USP <800>. However, because you have completed the Assessment of Risk and addressed the containment strategies and/or work practices you use, it may not have to be handled with all the containment strategies listed in USP <800>.

6.12 What antineoplastics don't have to be handled as HDs?

All antineoplastics need to be handled as HDs, but you may provide an entity exemption for specific dosage forms that have to be only counted or packaged. For example, conventionally manufactured fluorouracil cream is an antineoplastic, but if you need to only label it to dispense to a patient, it could be included in your Assessment of Risk. However, if you are compounding a fluorouracil cream for a patient-specific reason, it would need to be handled with all the containment strategies listed in <800>.

6.13 What about excluding "counting final dosage forms" when large quantity counting is performed?

Tablet and capsule forms of antineoplastic HDs cannot be placed in automated counting or packaging machines, because these could create powered contamination. Manual packaging of antineoplastic drugs is required. You could consider using automated equipment for the solid oral dosage forms of non-antineoplastics and reproductive hazards, but the risks would need to be identified and mitigated in your Assessment of Risk.

6.14 How often do I need to review the Assessment of Risk?

Review and document your Assessment of Risk at least every 12 months.

6.15 Who needs to know that I did an Assessment of Risk?

That depends on your state regulations, accreditation organization standards, and health-system policy. Consider reporting and documenting review of the Assessment of Risk at a medical staff committee meeting in a health system (e.g., the Pharmacy and Therapeutics Committee, Safety Committee). Have the document available for any survey or inspection in case it is requested.

6.16 What are some examples of alternative containment strategies?

Consider focusing on the dosage forms you handle. If you receive HDs in a final dosage form that is ready-for-administration (e.g., unit-dosed from the manufacturer or premixed infusions from a manufacturer or registered outsourcer), your exposure to potential contamination is limited. If you purchase premixed IV solutions from a manufacturer or outsourcing facility, your exposure to potential contamination is limited.

6.17 Would the containment strategies be applied to drugs (e.g., megestrol oral suspension) if the patient receives less than the full size of the unit dose?

If the nurse has to manipulate the drug, it isn't a ready-to-administer form. Antineoplastic agents that must be manipulated (e.g., a nurse pouring a liquid for a patient) need to be prepared under conditions that are compliant with <800>. Additionally, the Centers for Medicare & Medicaid Services (CMS) Hospital Conditions of Participation[9] and accreditation organization standards require that doses are provided in a ready-to-administer dosage form. Consider unit-dosing this in the pharmacy for patient-specific doses.

6.18 The NIOSH 2016 list of HDs says nurses must use double gloves for administration of anything on the HD list (even non-chemotherapy) except intact tablets or capsules. This seems excessive. Is this where the Assessment of Risk could be applied?

You need to use all the containment strategies for antineoplastic agents but could identify work practices in your Assessment of Risk to handle this situation. For example, you might want to include that a single pair of chemotherapy gloves (tested to American Society for Testing and Materials [ASTM] standard D6978) would be worn by the nurse administering any of the non-antineoplastics or reproductive hazards. Medication administration policies should address the containment strategies and work practices in your Assessment of Risk.

6.19 If I have to package methotrexate tablets, isn't the risk different for the tech who packages it versus the nurse who administers it?

It could be, and you can handle this in your Assessment of Risk. You might consider packaging the methotrexate tablets using a manual process in your biological safety cabinet (BSC) with all precautions listed in <800>. Once the tablets are contained in a unit-dose package, it would be a finished dosage form for nursing so it may not require the same level of containment precautions.

6.20 Do I have to exclude packaging and counting in my Assessment of Risk?

No, they need to be included. Assess this as part of your review for each drug and dosage form you handle.

6.21 What if I handle a non-antineoplastic HD but don't include it on my Assessment of Risk?

Then you need to follow all the containment strategies and work practices defined in <800>. Without the Assessment of Risk, the default requirement is to follow all containment precautions listed in <800>.

6.22 Can I do an Assessment of Risk for an entire class of drugs instead of listing each individual drug?

No. Your assessment of risk must list each drug and dosage form you handle. You might have the same information for several drugs or dosage forms, but your list needs to be specific to the drug and dosage form.

HUMAN RESOURCES 7

(See Sections 4, 8, 9, and 18 in USP <800>.)

7.1 MEDICAL SURVEILLANCE

7.1-1 What does *medical surveillance* mean?

Entities that handle hazardous drugs (HDs) should incorporate the standards in the Chapter into their occupational safety plan. Medical surveillance evaluates the protection provided by engineering controls, work practices, and personal protective equipment (PPE) as well as worker education concerning the materials exposed to during employment. The purpose is to minimize adverse health effects in personnel exposed to HDs. Medical surveillance programs include assessment and documentation of symptoms, physical findings, and laboratory studies to determine if there is deviation from expected norms. The National Institute of Occupational Safety and Health (NIOSH) document on *Medical Surveillance for Health Care Workers Exposed to Hazardous Drugs*[10] provides an overview.

7.1-2 What department determines how this will work?

This is an employee health issue, so there needs to be a system-wide policy concerning all healthcare personnel who may be exposed to HDs.

7.1-3 What types of medical surveillance will be required?

There is no requirement for medical surveillance; it is a recommendation. Of course, if your organization has specific policies, you are required to follow them. NIOSH has a document on medical surveillance available at http://www.cdc.gov/niosh/docs/wp-solutions/2013-103/pdfs/2013-103.pdf, and the Oncology Nursing Society (ONS) has excellent information in their publication *Safe Handling of Hazardous Drugs.*[11]

7.1-4 Should all employees have to sign lists acknowledging risk/NIOSH drug list?

Personnel of reproductive capability must confirm in writing that they understand the risks of handling HDs. This has been a requirement in <797> since 2008 and is required by <800>.

7.1-5 Should pregnant or breast-feeding pharmacy technicians and pharmacists, or any employees trying to conceive, be removed from work duties of preparing chemo?

This is an issue of employee health policies. NIOSH has published recommendations that may be helpful to review. See https://www.cdc.gov/niosh/docket/review/docket279/pdfs/alternativedutycibrevised12012014.pdf.

7.1-6 Should nurses who are pregnant or wish to become pregnant avoid taking care of patients who are on HDs due to administration and drug elimination in bodily fluids?

That is an issue your Employee Health and Risk Management leaders must determine. The NIOSH document on medical surveillance[10] and the ONS publication *Safe Handling of Hazardous Drugs*[11] are excellent resources.

7.2 DESIGNATED PERSON

> All entities must designate a specific individual who is responsible for overseeing activities handling HDs. This cannot be eliminated even if using the Assessment of Risk approach.

7.2-1 Who is the *designated person* mentioned in <800>?

Each entity—any site where HDs are handled—must have an individual who oversees the responsibilities of handling HDs. This person is responsible for developing and implementing policies and procedures; overseeing compliance with <800> and any other applicable laws, regulations, and standards; ensuring competency of personnel; and ensuring environmental control of the facilities used for storing and compounding HDs.

7.2-2 Can the *designated person* be a committee instead of an individual?

There needs to be a particular person identified. That person can lead a committee if that approach is chosen by the entity.

7.2-3 Does the *designated person* need to be a pharmacist?

No. It can be anyone qualified to perform all the required functions. Healthcare systems will most likely have a pharmacist in this position, but many entities (e.g., physician offices, veterinary clinics) may not have a pharmacist available for this function.

7.2-4 Does the *designated person* need to be a manager?

No. It is up to the entity to assign the specific person to oversee this.

7.2-5 Is the *designated person* responsible for compliance with USP <800>?

Yes, that is a key function of the designated person.

7.2-6 Does oversight of handling HDs have to be the *designated person's* sole job responsibility?

No. It is up to the entity to assign job functions.

7.2-7 Can the *designated person* be responsible for more than one site?

Yes. It is up to the entity to assign the responsibility. One person can have responsibility for multiple sites. In multihospital health systems, it is likely that one person would be responsible for oversight of multiple hospitals and other sites that handle HDs.

7.2-8 Where can the *designated person* obtain the necessary training for this job?

That is up to the entity to define. Training needs to include both didactic and hands-on experience. The requirements for training are defined in <800>, and references in the appendix to <800> can be used as sources.

7.2-9 How much training does the *designated person* need to have?

<800> does not specify the number of hours. Some state regulations require a specific number for re-licensure of pharmacists and/or other compounders. The designated person must have a thorough understanding of the standards to be able to develop, implement, and oversee policies, procedures, and practices including personnel training, evaluation, and monitoring as well as facility compliance with <800> and other laws and regulations.

7.3 RESPONSIBILITIES OF COMPOUNDING PERSONNEL TRAINING

7.3-1 What training is required to handle HDs?

Education and training concerning HDs need to supplement general education, training, and documentation of competency for handling any drug. *Competence Assessment Tools for Health-System Pharmacies*[12] provides checklists and competence documents, including one for compounding HDs (see **Appendix**); <795> and <797> have sections concerning personnel training specific to compounding. All personnel handling HDs need to complete some HD training such as identifying HDs, organizational policies and procedures, use of PPE, use of engineering controls and other devices, response to exposure to HDs, spill management, and proper disposal of HDs. Employees such as those who only unpack orders and deliver finished HD preparations or environmental services personnel need information targeted to their duties. Personnel performing specific functions, such as compounding or administering, require additional training targeted to those activities. Personnel must document competency prior to independently handling HDs. Personnel training must occur before a new HD or new equipment is used, and competency must be documented at least every 12 months.

7.4 DOCUMENTING COMPETENCE

7.4-1 What competence information has to be documented?

Competence documents should show that the person can perform functions of the position and that they will comply with your organizational policies and procedures. *Competence Assessment Tools for Health-System Pharmacies*[12] provides compounding- and HD-related assessments and forms. Compounding requires observation by skilled personnel to ensure proper techniques are followed; be sure to document this observational review and approval.

7.4-2 How often should training occur?

Initial training needs to meet the requirements of <795> and/or <797> as well as the HD-specific information in <800>. Ongoing education and training need to occur whenever new HDs or new equipment is used. Documentation of ongoing competence needs to occur at least every 12 months.

7.4-3 If we add a new drug similar to one we use, does that require full annual-type documentation?

Not necessarily. This depends on your organizational policy. In some cases, an in-service related to the new drug and compounding and administration requirements might be sufficient. You would also need to update your HD list with this new information.

7.4-4 Who needs to be trained on the hazards of HDs?

Anyone who handles them must be trained. There needs to be general training for anyone handling HDs including receiving personnel, those involved in storage and transport of HDs, compounding personnel, nurses, and others who administer HDs as well as environmental services personnel who handle waste. Specific functions—receiving, compounding, administering, etc.—must have additional targeted training particular to their functions.

7.4-5 Do I still need to do the personnel training listed in <795>?

Yes. All the training information in <795> must be followed for those who compound nonsterile HD preparations.

7.4-6 Do I still need to do the personnel training listed in <797>?

Yes. All the training in <797> must be done for those who compound sterile HD preparations.

7.4-7 Does <800> require training separate from what we do for the hospital?

There is no separate training required as long as your training includes all of the elements listed in <800>. The training that you do needs to be targeted to the duties the employee will perform.

7.4-8 Do I need to teach my night nursing supervisors how to use the chemo hood?

No. There is no reason that a hospital nursing supervisor should have to work in any primary engineering control (PEC) if a pharmacy is on site. If antineoplastic HD compounded sterile preparations are needed in a hospital, personnel with documented competency for the task must prepare them under <797>- and <800>-compliant conditions. If the hospital's Assessment of Risk allows preparation of those HDs that are not antineoplastic under urgent circumstances outside of a C-PEC, no PEC is needed because it should be only for a single dose that would be immediately administered.

7.5 HAZARD COMMUNICATION PLAN

All entities must have a Hazard Communication Plan. This is an OSHA requirement, and it cannot be eliminated even if using the Assessment of Risk approach.

7.5-1 What is a Hazard Communication Plan?

The Occupational Safety and Health Administration (OSHA) requires all workplaces where employees are exposed to hazardous chemicals to have a written plan describing how the standard will be implemented in that facility. See https://www.osha.gov/dsg/hazcom/solutions.html.

7.5-2 Whose responsibility is it to develop a Hazard Communication Plan?

In a health system, this will be a function of the Safety Department or other assigned responsibility. For small employers that need a summary document, see OSHA's Hazard Communication: *Small Entity Compliance Guide for Employers That Use Hazardous Chemicals* at https://www.osha.gov/Publications/OSHA3695.pdf.

7.5-3 Is a hazardous chemical the same thing as a HD?

Not necessarily. The HDs defined in <800> are those in the NIOSH list of HDs.[5] OSHA's hazardous chemical standard includes much more than the NIOSH list, since it deals with all types of hazardous chemicals, not just those that are hazardous to healthcare personnel.

7.5-4 Do all HDs require a Safety Data Sheet (SDS)?

The OSHA Hazard Communication Standard exempts final forms of U.S. Food and Drug Administration (FDA)-approved drugs when in solid final form (e.g., tablets, pills) for direct administration to the patient. See https://www.osha.gov/pls/oshaweb/owadisp.show_document?p_table=INTERPRETATIONS&p_id=21231.

7.5-5 What are the occupational exposure limits for HDs?

There is currently no standard for acceptable limits for HD exposure.

7.5-6 Do employees have to document that they know they are working with HDs?

<800> requires personnel of reproductive capability to confirm in writing that they understand the risks of handling HDs. This has been a requirement of USP <797> since 2008 and is also included in <800>.

7.5-7 Do both male and female employees need to document their acknowledgment of HDs?

Yes.

7.5-8 Where can I get an example of an employee consent form regarding exposure to HDs?

See **Exhibit** 7-1 for a sample of an acknowledgment of HD risk form.

EXHIBIT 7-1 Sample Acknowledgment of Hazardous Drug Risk

Name of Employee: _____

I understand working with or near hazardous drugs in healthcare settings may cause skin rashes, infertility, miscarriage, birth defects, and possibly leukemia or other cancers.

I understand that Sample Pharmacy maintains detailed policies and procedures on the proper storage, handling, transport, and disposal of hazardous drugs. Sample Pharmacy has put in place a variety of administrative, engineering, and work practice controls to reduce the risk of occupational exposure to hazardous drugs. I understand Sample Pharmacy's policies and procedures will be amended on an annual basis, and the policies and procedures seek to reflect information, standards, and regulations from relevant local, state, and federal regulatory bodies as well as practice standards from professional associations.

I have been provided with didactic training that reflects the policies and procedures on hazardous drugs and have been afforded the opportunity to ask questions. After completion of the training I have been required to take and successfully pass written testing and have also had my hazardous drug handling techniques observed and documented on the Hazardous Drug Competency. Retraining and competency evaluation will occur annually. I received and successfully completed this training prior to performing any activity associated with hazardous drugs. I understand Sample Pharmacy's policies and procedures and agree to abide by them at all times. I also agree that I will immediately seek out the Pharmacy Manager or my direct supervisor should a question occur during work activities.

I acknowledge that failure to follow the established policies and procedures may put me at risk of exposure to hazardous substances which can lead to acute effects such as skin rashes; chronic effects, including adverse reproductive events such as infertility, miscarriage, or birth defects; and possibly the development of cancer.

_____   _____
Signature of Employee Name above   Date

Source: ©1997-2016 Clinical IQ, LLC. All rights reserved. Used with permission.

PERSONAL PROTECTIVE EQUIPMENT 8

(See Section 7 in USP <800>.)

PPE listed in <800> must be used for handling API of any type of hazardous drug and for antineoplastic agents. The entity's policies and procedures must list the requirements in addition to what is listed in <800> as requirements.

8.1 GENERAL INFORMATION

8.1-1 What does <800> require for PPE?

Depending on the activities performed, <800> requires chemotherapy gloves tested to meet American Society for Testing and Materials (ASTM) standard D6978; gowns that are long-sleeved impermeable and close in the back (no opening in the front) and have closed cuffs that are elastic or knit; hair covers; beard covers; shoe covers; face and eye protection; and respiratory protection.

8.1-2 What are the benefits of PPE?

Personal protective equipment (PPE) limits the amount of exposure to hazardous drug (HD) aerosols and particles.

8.1-3 Are all the components of PPE needed for every activity when handling HDs?

Not necessarily. Different functions have different PPE requirements. See the National Institute for Occupational Safety and Health (NIOSH) list of HDs[7] for recommended PPE based on the activity performed.

8.1-4 What does *donning* and *doffing* mean?

Don means to put on PPE; ***doff*** means to remove it.

8.1-5 What does *hand hygiene* mean?

The Centers for Disease Control and Prevention (CDC) defines *hand hygiene* as "cleaning your hands by using either handwashing (washing hands with soap and water), antiseptic hand wash, antiseptic hand rub (i.e., alcohol-based hand sanitizer including foam or gel), or surgical hand antisepsis." For HD handling, you need to wash your hands with soap and water because the mechanical process of rubbing your hands together helps to remove any HD contamination. Use of only hand rubs is not sufficient to remove HD contamination. See the CDC Hand Hygiene Guideline at www.cdc.gov/handhygiene for further information.

8.1-6 When gloves are mentioned in <800>, does that mean *chemo gloves*?

Yes. *Gloves* means chemotherapy gloves that have been tested to meet ASTM standard D6978.

8.1-7 What PPE needs to be worn by receiving personnel?

<800> requires use of chemotherapy gloves when unpacking HDs. Many personnel in receiving areas wear work gloves; if these are worn, the work gloves should be over the chemotherapy gloves. If the items received are not enclosed in plastic, <800> recommends wearing an elastomeric half-mask with a multi-gas cartridge and P100 filter until the packaging can be checked to be sure it is not damaged. Protective gowns and respiratory protection are needed if spills or leaks occur, and a spill kit must be available in the receiving area.

The entity's policies and procedures must describe the appropriate PPE to be worn based on its occupational safety plan, which must address the risk of exposure and activities performed. See the PPE recommendations in the NIOSH list of HDs[5] and the NIOSH Workplace Solutions document *Personal Protective Equipment for Health Care Workers Who Work with Hazardous Drugs*[13] for additional information.

If the entity has performed an Assessment of Risk and identified alternative containment strategies and/or work practices for agents that are listed in the NIOSH HD list as non-antineoplastic or reproductive hazards, those strategies and work practices concerning PPE may differ from the requirements for antineoplastic agents or active pharmaceutical ingredients (APIs).

Also see information under Section 9, Receiving Personnel: Hazardous Drug Precautions.

8.1-8 What PPE needs to be worn by personnel who are transporting HDs?

<800> doesn't specify the PPE requirements for transporting HDs, but similar protection as used for receiving is logical. Those transporting HDs should use chemotherapy gloves. Protective gowns and respiratory protection are needed if spills or leaks occur, and a spill kit should be accessible.

The entity's policies and procedures must describe the appropriate PPE to be worn based on its occupational safety plan, which must address the risk of exposure and activities performed. See the PPE recommendations in the NIOSH list of HDs[5] and the NIOSH Workplace Solutions document *Personal Protective Equipment for Health Care Workers Who Work with Hazardous Drugs*[13] for additional information.

If the entity has performed an Assessment of Risk and identified alternative containment strategies and/or work practices for agents that are listed in the NIOSH HD list as non-antineoplastic or reproductive hazards, those strategies and work practices concerning PPE may differ from the requirements for antineoplastic agents or APIs.

8.1-9 What PPE needs to be worn by personnel who are packaging HDs?

Personnel who are unit-dose packaging oral HDs that are not intact (e.g., those containers with broken tablets or extraneous powder) require similar PPE as used for compounding: chemotherapy gloves, impervious gown, hair covers, shoe covers, and, if not packaging the agents in a containment primary engineering control (C-PEC), eye and respiratory protection.

The entity's policies and procedures must describe the appropriate PPE to be worn based on its occupational safety plan, which must address the risk of exposure and activities performed. See the PPE recommendations in the NIOSH list of HDs[5] and the NIOSH Workplace Solutions document *Personal Protective Equipment for Health Care Workers Who Work with Hazardous Drugs*[13] for additional information.

Packaging undamaged oral HDs that require only counting and placement in a prescription vial may be evaluated under the entity's Assessment of Risk. For antineoplastic agents, use of chemotherapy gloves and equipment (e.g., counting trays, spatulas) that are dedicated to use with antineoplastics should be considered.

If the entity has performed an Assessment of Risk and identified alternative containment strategies and/or work practices for agents that are listed in the NIOSH HD list as antineoplastics, or agents that are listed in the NIOSH HD list as non-antineoplastic or reproductive hazards, those strategies and work practices concerning PPE may differ from the requirements for antineoplastic agents or APIs.

Also see information under Section 18, Dispensing Hazardous Drugs.

8.1-10 What PPE needs to be worn by personnel who are compounding HDs?

Two pairs of chemotherapy gloves, an impervious gown designed for use with HDs, hair covers, beard covers, and shoe covers are required for nonsterile and sterile HD compounding. If compounding a compounded sterile preparation (CSP), a surgical mask is required to protect the CSP from microbial contamination. If working outside of a C-PEC (e.g., preparation in the surgical suite), eye and respiratory protection is needed.

The entity's policies and procedures must describe the appropriate PPE to be worn based on its occupational safety plan, which must address the risk of exposure and activities performed. See the PPE recommendations in the NIOSH list of HDs[5] and the NIOSH Workplace Solutions document *Personal Protective Equipment for Health Care Workers Who Work with Hazardous Drugs*[13] for additional information.

If the entity has performed an Assessment of Risk and identified alternative containment strategies and/or work practices for agents that are listed in the NIOSH HD list as non-antineoplastic or reproductive hazards, those strategies and work practices concerning PPE may differ from the requirements for antineoplastic agents or APIs.

Also see information under Section 15, Compounding Hazardous Drugs.

8.1-11 Does the pharmacist checking the preparation compounded in the C-PEC need to wear all PPE if he or she is not touching anything, but just looking?

Anyone inside the negative pressure room or in the anteroom needs to be appropriately garbed. Checking an intravenous (IV) involves more than just looking at it. The integrity of the final preparation and container needs to be assessed. See USP <797> for more information.

8.1-12 If a pharmacist completes the checking of a CSP in the anteroom, does he or she need to garb?

Anyone inside the negative pressure room or anteroom needs to be appropriately garbed. Checking an IV involves more than just looking at it. The integrity of the final preparation and container needs to be assessed. See USP <797> for more information.

8.1-13 Is additional PPE required for personnel who are compounding from powders?

This should be considered in your Assessment of Risk and PPE policies and practices. There is certainly an eye and respiratory risk when working with APIs and other raw materials.

8.1-14 My CACI technical manual states that head/hair/shoe covers are not required when compounding. Does USP supersede that?

Yes. You need to wear the PPE when working with HDs in a compounding aseptic containment isolator (CACI). The PPE is to protect you as the compounder.

8.1-15 Should PPE be donned before entering the negative pressure lab?

In a sterile compounding suite, don the PPE in the positive pressure anteroom prior to entering the negative pressure buffer room. In a containment segregated compounding area (C-SCA) or nonsterile HD room, don the PPE outside the perimeter line around the C-PEC.

8.1-16 Is it necessary for the compounding pharmacist to remove all PPE each time he or she steps out to answer the phone?

Yes. PPE exposed in the negative pressure areas needs to be removed just prior to exiting the room. You would be exposing all personnel and patients to potential HD contamination by wearing the PPE outside the negative pressure room.

8.1-17 The compounding pharmacist does all the patient counseling when new prescriptions are picked up. Does the pharmacist have to remove all PPE each time during the day when counseling a patient?

Yes. PPE exposed in the negative pressure areas needs to be removed just prior to exiting the room. You would be exposing all personnel and patients to potential HD contamination by wearing the PPE outside the negative pressure room.

8.1-18 Is an N95 respirator required when compounding HDs that could cause a respiratory risk?

If respiratory protection is required, an N95 or P100 device should be used. A simple surgical mask is not adequate. N95 and most other respiratory protective devices require fit-testing for each employee who would use them.

8.1-19 How do PPE requirements differ between nonsterile and sterile compounding?

The same PPE requirements apply whether the compounding is for nonsterile or sterile preparations. The only difference is the requirement for gloves to be sterile when compounding sterile preparations.

8.1-20 Do you have to wear PPE when transporting drugs to an infusion area?

Yes. The specific requirements need to be included in your policy. See the PPE recommendations in the NIOSH list of HDs[5] and the NIOSH Workplace Solutions document *Personal Protective Equipment for Health Care Workers Who Work with Hazardous Drugs*[13] for additional information.

8.1-21 What PPE needs to be worn by personnel who are administering HDs?

For administering parenteral antineoplastics, two pairs of chemotherapy gloves are required. For administering parenteral antineoplastics, an impervious gown intended for use with HDs is also required. If splashing is possible, eye protection is needed. If the potential of inhaling HDs is present, respiratory protection is needed.

The entity's policies and procedures must describe the appropriate PPE to be worn based on its occupational safety plan, which must address the risk of exposure and activities performed. See the PPE recommendations in the NIOSH list of HDs[5] and the NIOSH Workplace Solutions document *Personal Protective Equipment for Health Care Workers Who Work with Hazardous Drugs*[13] for additional information.

If the entity has performed an Assessment of Risk and identified alternative containment strategies and/or work practices for agents that are listed in the NIOSH HD list as non-antineoplastic or reproductive hazards, those strategies and work practices concerning PPE may differ from the requirements for antineoplastic agents or APIs.

Also see information under Section 20, Administering Hazardous Drugs.

8.1-22 What PPE needs to be worn by personnel who are discarding HD trash?

Personnel disposing of HD trash should wear chemotherapy gloves and an impervious gown intended for use with HDs. If splashing is possible, eye protection is needed. If the potential of inhaling HDs is present, respiratory protection is needed.

The entity's policies and procedures must describe the appropriate PPE to be worn based on its occupational safety plan, which must address the risk of exposure and activities performed. See the PPE recommendations in the NIOSH list of HDs[5] and the NIOSH Workplace Solutions document *Personal Protective Equipment for Health Care Workers Who Work with Hazardous Drugs*[13] for additional information.

If the entity has performed an Assessment of Risk and identified alternative containment strategies and/or work practices for agents that are listed in the NIOSH HD list as non-antineoplastic or reproductive hazards, those strategies and work practices concerning PPE may differ from the requirements for antineoplastic agents or APIs.

8.1-23 What PPE does personnel need to wear when cleaning up a spill?

Personnel cleaning up a spill should wear chemotherapy gloves, an impervious gown intended for use with HDs, hair cover, shoe covers, goggles, and a fit-tested full-facepiece as well as chemical cartridge-type respirator or powered air-purifying respirator (PAPR).

The entity's policies and procedures must describe the appropriate PPE to be worn based on its occupational safety plan, which must address the risk of exposure and activities performed. See the PPE recommendations in the NIOSH list of HDs[5] and the NIOSH Workplace Solutions document *Personal Protective Equipment for Health Care Workers Who Work with Hazardous Drugs*[13] for additional information.

If the entity has performed an Assessment of Risk and identified alternative containment strategies and/or work practices for agents that are listed in the NIOSH HD list as non-antineoplastic or reproductive hazards, those strategies and work practices concerning PPE may differ from the requirements for antineoplastic agents or APIs.

Also see information under Section 24, Spills.

8.1-24 Can PPE be reused?

Disposable PPE must not be reused. Reusable PPE must be decontaminated and cleaned after use.

8.1-25 What is meant by "reused"? Can garb be reused if removed and then donned again when required to leave the area for just a few minutes? Or does it mean reused on a different day?

Garb exposed to HDs must be removed and disposable components discarded when leaving the negative pressure area, even for just a few minutes. It cannot be hung inside or outside the compounding area and then used again.

8.1-26 Is PPE required when using a compounding isolator?

Yes. The same PPE is required with either a biological safety cabinet (BSC) or CACI.

8.1-27 <797> allows use of a gown throughout one shift. Does this apply when compounding HDs?

No. Disposable PPE used for HD compounding must not be reused.

8.1-28 Does the pharmacist who is checking only items need to garb?

Anyone within the negative pressure room or ante area needs to garb.

8.1-29 What is the proper order of donning and doffing PPE for compounding HDs in a cleanroom suite (positive pressure anteroom and negative pressure buffer room)?

To don PPE:

1. Enter dirty side of positive pressure anteroom.
2. Don mask, hair cover, two pairs of shoe covers.
3. Step over into clean side of anteroom.
4. Wash hands.
5. Don gown followed by chemo gown.
6. Apply alcohol-based hand rub with persistent antimicrobial activity.
7. Don two pairs of sterile chemo gloves—one under the cuff of the gown, and one over the cuff of the gown.

To doff PPE:

1. Remove outer pair of chemo gloves prior to handling the container (e.g., chemo bag) the preparation will be placed into.
2. Just prior to leaving the negative pressure buffer area, remove chemo gown and outer pair of shoe covers.
3. Remove all garb when leaving the anteroom.

8.1-30 What is the proper order of donning and doffing PPE for compounding HDs in a C-SCA?

To don PPE:

1. Enter C-SCA.
2. Don mask, hair cover, two pairs of shoe covers.
3. Wash hands.
4. Don chemo gown.
5. Apply alcohol-based hand rub with persistent antimicrobial activity.
6. Don two pairs of sterile chemo gloves—one under the cuff of the gown, and one over the cuff of the gown.

To doff PPE:

1. Remove outer pair of chemo gloves prior to handling the container (e.g., chemo bag) the preparation will be placed into.
2. Just prior to leaving the negative pressure area, remove chemo gown and outer pair of shoe covers.
3. Remove all garb when compounding session is complete.

What is the proper order of donning and doffing PPE for compounding HDs in a compounding room for nonsterile HD preparation?

To don PPE:

1. Enter negative pressure compounding room.
2. Don mask, hair cover, two pairs of shoe covers.
3. Wash hands.
4. Don chemo gown.
5. Apply alcohol-based hand rub with persistent antimicrobial activity.
6. Don two pairs of chemo gloves—one under the cuff of the gown, and one over the cuff of the gown.

To doff PPE:

1. Remove outer pair of chemo gloves prior to handling transport container (e.g., chemo bag) the preparation will be placed into.
2. Just prior to leaving the negative pressure area, remove chemo gown and outer pair of shoe covers.
3. Remove all garb when compounding session is completed.

8.2 GLOVES

8.2-1 Do chemo gloves have to meet a particular standard?

Yes. Gloves used for handling HDs must meet ASTM Standard D6978, the *Standard Practice for Assessment of Resistance of Medical Gloves to Permeation by Chemotherapy Drugs.*[14] Some gloves are tested only for permeation to general chemicals using ASTM Standard F739-99a (*Standard Test Method for Resistance of Protective Clothing Materials to Permeation by Liquids or Gases under Conditions of Continuous Contact*[15]), which is not sufficient for HD gloves.

8.2-2 How do I know if a glove is chemo-rated?

Documentation that the gloves meet ASTM 6978 needs to be listed on the product label. It can generally be found on the box of the gloves.

8.2-3 Is it OK for chemo gloves to be tested per ASTM D6978 and lab chemical tested per ASTM F739?

Yes, as long as they document that they meet the ASTM Standard D6978.

8.2-4 Do I have to wear chemo gloves when handling non-antineoplastic HDs?

That would need to be defined in your entity's Assessment of Risk. The labeling for many general medical gloves document that they meet ASTM 6978, so there are options for glove products meeting the chemotherapy glove standard even if they are not sterile nor designed specifically for HD use.

8.2-5 Do sterile chemo gloves exist?

Yes. Sterile chemo gloves are available from a variety of suppliers.

8.2-6 When must you use sterile gloves?

Sterile gloves must be used when you are compounding a sterile preparation.

8.2-7 How do I sterilize chemo gloves?

For compounding CSPs, you need to use sterile chemotherapy gloves. For disinfecting gloves during compounding, use sterile 70% isopropyl alcohol (sIPA) applied by using a sterile wipe saturated with sIPA. Do not spray alcohol (or any other solution) in a HD area because that could aerosolize the HD.

8.2-8 Is double-gloving required?

In most cases, the answer is yes. A single chemotherapy glove is acceptable when administering an intact tablet or capsule. Otherwise, two pairs of chemotherapy gloves are required.

8.2-9 Why do I need to wear two pairs of gloves?

After compounding, you need to remove the outer glove so you can handle and label the completed compound without contaminating it with hazardous residue. For all instances where two gloves are required, the inner glove is a redundant barrier if the outer glove is torn or punctured or must be removed because of contamination.

8.2-10 How can you put on two pairs of gloves? They don't fit over each other.

Consider using a half-size larger glove for the outer glove.

8.2-11 Can the inner glove be a regular glove and the outer glove be a chemo glove?

No. When two pairs of gloves are required, two pairs of chemotherapy gloves that meet ASTM standard D6978 are needed.

8.2-12 Are chemo gloves required when working in a compounding isolator?

Yes, working in either a BSC or a CACI requires the same PPE.

8.2-13 Do I need two pairs of chemo gloves if I'm working inside a CACI?

Yes. You need two pairs of chemotherapy gloves that meet ASTM standard D6978. You may also use or need to use another pair of gloves to meet the CACI operating procedure.

8.2-14 We use a CACI. Is the isolator glove considered to be the second pair of gloves, or do we need two pairs plus the isolator glove?

It depends on the design of your CACI gauntlet and glove assembly. In any case, you need two pairs of chemotherapy gloves that meet ASTM standard D6978. You may also use or need to use another pair of gloves to meet the CACI operating procedure.

8.2-15 Do both pairs of chemo gloves need to be sterile?

That depends on the activity being performed. If you are working in a BSC or CACI, use two pairs of sterile gloves because you will need to remove the outer pair prior to labeling the CSP. The inner glove needs to be sterile in this case, since you will be working within a C-PEC.

8.2-16 Do both pairs of gloves need to be made of the same material?

Both pairs of gloves need to meet the ASTM standard D6978 but do not necessarily need to be the same material.

8.2-17 How often do gloves need to be changed?

Change the chemotherapy gloves every 30 minutes unless otherwise recommended by the manufacturer's documentation. The gloves must be changed if they are torn or punctured or if you know or suspect they have been contaminated.

8.2-18 Where do I find the manufacturer's information about the glove permeability?

Most manufacturers place the glove permeability information on the box of gloves.

8.2-19 How do I find a glove that I can use with carmustine or thiotepa?

Manufacturers test the gloves against certain HDs. Different drugs have different permeation time. Some drugs permeate different materials at different rates. Check with the manufacturers to see if they have information in addition to what is listed on their product labeling.

8.3 GOWNS

8.3-1 Do chemo gowns have to meet a particular standard?

No, unfortunately there is no standard test for chemotherapy gowns.

8.3-2 How do I know if a gown is chemo-rated?

There is no standard test, so you have to depend on the manufacturer's labeling. A gown used for handling HDs needs to be disposable and resist permeation by HDs. Some manufacturers provide results of drug-specific permeation tests. Others use an ASTM standard—but not the same as the glove standard—for permeation of drugs through their gowns.[15]

8.3-3 What documentation exists concerning permeability of chemo gowns?

Obtain that information from the gown manufacturer.

8.3-4 How do I know that a particular gown will resist permeability to HDs?

Some manufacturers use the ASTM standard F739[15] to test their gowns. Obtain the information from the gown manufacturer.

8.3-5 What is the difference between gowns we use for non-HDs and those used for chemo?

Gowns used for handling antineoplastic agents must be impervious. Gowns used for non-HDs can be made of other materials, depending on their intended use. Your entity's Assessment of Risk may allow different gowns when handling non-antineoplastic or reproductive hazard HDs.

8.3-6 What are chemo gowns supposed to be made of?

Many chemotherapy gowns are made of polyethylene-coated polypropylene or a similar laminate material.

8.3-7 How should chemo gowns be constructed?

Gowns must be disposable, seamless, and close in the back (no open front); have long sleeves; and have cuffs that are made of elastic or a knit material.

8.3-8 In pharmacy, we have blue plastic gowns for mixing chemo. Our nurses wear yellow isolation gowns when they administer chemo. Is this OK?

As long as the pharmacy gowns are impervious and intended for handling HDs, you are using the correct gown in the pharmacy. The ***nursing gown is NOT OK:*** the yellow gowns commonly used as isolation gowns in hospitals provide no protection against contamination from HDs. Nursing needs to use gowns that comply with the requirements in <800>.

8.3-9 Can I hang my gown in the anteroom for use later in the day?

No. Disposable PPE cannot be reused. You need to discard it in the buffer room or the C-SCA prior to leaving that area to avoid contaminating the anteroom or other area.

8.3-10 <797> allows a gown to be removed, retained, and used throughout the work shift if it isn't soiled. Is this allowed by <800>?

No. PPE exposed in handling HDs is potentially contaminated with HD residue, so it cannot be reused.

8.3-11 Can gowns be re-worn during the day if a compounder must leave the HD compounding area? How should it be removed, stored, and re-donned?

The gowns cannot be saved for future use, even within the same shift. They must be discarded when leaving the negative pressure area.

8.3-12 Are washable gowns allowed?

No, washable gowns are not allowed for handling antineoplastic HDs. Your entity's Assessment of Risk may allow washable gowns for non-antineoplastics or reproductive hazards.

8.3-13 If we use a reusable gown service and their cleaning procedures are sufficient, does that qualify as disposable?

No. Gowns must be disposable.

8.3-14 How often do gowns need to be changed?

Gowns must be changed based on the manufacturer's information for permeation of the gown. If no permeation information is available for the gowns used, change them every 2-3 hours or immediately after a spill or splash.

8.3-15 How long can I use a chemo gown—one compound, one batch, or all day?

Gowns must be changed based on the manufacturer's information for permeation of the gown. If no permeation information is available for the gowns used, change them every 2-3 hours or immediately after a spill or splash. As you leave the negative pressure room (either the buffer room of the cleanroom suite or the C-SCA), you must remove and discard the gown; it cannot be saved for use later.

8.3-16 Why do I have to change my gown every 2-3 hours?

This information has been in the *ASHP Guidelines on Handling Hazardous Drugs*[3] for years, and it has also been in other guidance documents. There is no ASTM standard for permeation of HDs through gowns, so you need to rely on the manufacturer's information. If no permeation information is available, change them every 2-3 hours. Of course, if there is a spill, you need to change the gown right away.

8.3-17 Do I need to wear a regular gown under my chemo gown?

That is not specified in <800>, but you should think about your facility design and work practices. If you are in a sterile compounding suite, you need to have a regular gown under your chemo gown since you will be entering the clean side of your anteroom when you exit your negative pressure buffer room. You have to be properly gowned at that point, so you need to have on a gown, gloves, mask, hair cover, and shoe covers.

If your HD facility is a C-SCA or an area devoted to nonsterile compounding, you may not need a regular gown because you will be exiting into a general pharmacy area. However, think of your containment practices. Consider using a regular gown even in these situations to further protect your clothing.

8.3-18 Do two gowns always need to be worn when compounding or is one chemo gown OK?

That is not specified in <800>, but you should think about your facility design and work practices. If you are in a sterile compounding suite, you need to have a regular gown under your chemo gown because you will be entering the clean side of your anteroom when you exit your negative pressure buffer room. You have to be properly gowned at that point, so you need to have on a gown, gloves, mask, hair cover, and shoe covers.

If your HD facility is a C-SCA or an area devoted to nonsterile compounding, you may not need a regular gown since you will be exiting into a general pharmacy area. However, think of your containment practices. Consider using a regular gown even in these situations to further protect your clothing.

8.4 HAIR COVERS

8.4-1 What is the difference between head and beard covers used for chemo and those used for non-HDs?

There is no difference. The same products can be used for handling HDs as you use for handling non-HDs.

8.4-2 If personnel wear a head cover for religious or other reasons, is an additional hair cover necessary?

Yes. The purpose of the hair covers is to protect the preparation from potential microbial contamination and to protect personnel from transferring potential HD contamination to other areas. Hair covers come in various formats, including bouffants and hoods. The additional hair covers must be placed over the head cover worn for religious or other reasons.

8.5 SHOE COVERS

8.5-1 What is the difference between shoe covers used for chemo and those used for non-HDs?

There is no difference. The same products can be used for handling HDs as you use for handling non-HDs. However, you may want to consider using shoe covers that are impervious.

8.5-2 Can I use dedicated cleanroom shoes instead of shoe covers?

No, you need to use shoe covers even if you have dedicated shoes for your cleanroom.

8.5-3 Why does <800> require two pairs of shoe covers?

The floor in front of the BSC or CACI is one of the most likely places where HD contamination could be found. You need to have on two pairs of shoe covers so you can remove the outer pair prior to entering the anteroom or C-SCA to avoid tracking contamination into other areas.

8.5-4 Do nurses need to wear shoe covers when administering chemo?

Shoe covers are not required by <800> when administering HDs, but you should consider this additional precaution in your Assessment of Risk and garbing policies.

8.6 EYE PROTECTION

8.6-1 What does *eye protection* mean?

When eye protection is needed, it needs to be provided by using goggles. Goggles fit tightly, covering the eyes, eye sockets, and facial area surrounding the eyes. Goggles can be obtained that fit over eye glasses.

8.6-2 Do I need goggles if I wear glasses?

Yes. Eyeglasses don't protect your entire eye socket area.

8.6-3 When is eye protection needed?

You need to have eye protection—goggles—when there is a risk of spills or splashes. In particular, wear eye protection when you are working with HDs outside of a C-PEC, for administration of HDs in the Operating Suite, when you are working with HDs above eye level, or cleaning up a spill.

8.6-4 I wear prescription eyeglasses. Does this qualify as eye protection?

No. Eyeglasses alone do not protect against splashes to the eyes. You need to obtain goggles that fit over your eyeglasses.

8.6-5 I wear a face shield when I mix chemo. Is this proper eye protection?

No. Face shields alone do not protect against splashes to the eyes. You have to wear goggles when eye protection is needed. However, you don't necessarily need to use additional eye protection when working in a BSC or CACI unless your organizational policy requires it.

8.6-6 Do I need eye protection when I'm mixing chemo?

A BSC with the sash down in the proper position and a CACI provide eye protection, so normal operation may not require additional eye protection. However, you need to have eye protection if there is a risk of spills or splashes. Those situations where HDs are being manipulated outside a C-PEC (e.g., patient administration in the Operating Suite) require eye protection, since you don't have the protection of the C-PEC in that case.

8.6-7 Do I need eye protection when I'm cleaning the area inside a BSC or CACI?

If splashing is possible, you need eye protection.

8.6-8 Do I need eye protection when I'm cleaning HD areas outside a C-PEC?

If splashing is possible, you need eye protection.

8.6-9 Do I need eye protection when I'm cleaning up a spill?

Yes. Wear eye protection when cleaning up a spill.

8.7 RESPIRATORY PROTECTION

8.7-1 What does *respiratory protection* mean?

When respiratory protection is needed, fit-tested NIOSH-certified N95 or more protective respirator is generally adequate to protect against airborne particles. However, N95 respirators don't protect against gases or vapors and provide only limited protection against direct liquid splashes. See the NIOSH page on Respiratory Trusted-Source Information at http://www.cdc.gov/niosh/npptl/topics/respirators/disp_part/respsource.html for more information.

8.7-2 What does an N95 respirator protect against?

It provides protection against airborne particles. It does not protect against gases or vapors.

8.7-3 Are there respirators that are better protection than N95?

There are other respirators that may meet your needs, which you should determine at your organization. Other types include full-facepiece, chemical cartridge-type respirators, elastomeric half-mask respirators with multi-gas cartridges and P100 filters (or a cartridge targeted to the specific drug), or PAPRs.

8.7-4 When is respiratory protection needed?

Respiratory protection is needed when there is known or suspected airborne exposure to particles or vapors, such as

- receiving HDs that are not contained in plastic until the integrity of the package can be confirmed;
- working outside of a C-PEC (e.g., for administration of HDs in the Operating Suite);
- cleaning under the work surface of a C-PEC; or
- cleaning up a spill.

8.7-5 Do I need respiratory protection when I'm working in a BSC or CACI?

The BSC or CACI provides respiratory protection when you are working in them, so no additional respiratory protection is needed unless the drug or procedure requires it. When compounding sterile preparations, you need to wear a mask (as you would during any sterile compounding); the mask is for protection of the preparation, not for your respiratory protection.

8.7-6 Do surgical masks provide adequate respiratory protection?

Surgical masks do not provide respiratory protection from drug exposure and must not be used alone when respiratory protection from HD exposure is required.

8.7-7 Since the BSC and CACI provide respiratory protection, do I need to wear a regular mask for any HD compounding?

You need a regular mask when compounding any sterile preparation, including HDs. Also consider use of a mask to protect nonsterile preparations. The regular (surgical) mask in this situation is for protection of the preparation you are mixing.

...nel need to wear respiratory protection when

...king HDs that are not contained in plastic should wear an elastomeric ... cartridge and P100 filter until assessment of the packaging integrity ... no spillage or breakage occurred during transport. If the type of drug ... more targeted cartridge can be used.

8.7-9 ... a surgical mask when compounding?

A surgical mask is required for sterile compounding and recommended for nonsterile compounding. However, a surgical mask is *not* respiratory protection; it protects the preparation, not the compounder.

8.7-10 Do I need to wear a respirator when I'm mixing chemo?

A BSC with the sash down in the proper position and a CACI provide respiratory protection, so normal operation may not require a respirator. Those situations where HDs are being manipulated outside a C-PEC (e.g., patient administration in the Operating Suite) require respiratory protection because you don't have the protection of the C-PEC in that case.

8.7-11 Can a surgical N95 respirator be used in place of a regular N95 respirator?

Yes. A surgical N95 respirator combines the respiratory protection of an N95 respirator and the protection of a surgical mask.

8.7-12 Does everyone who works with HDs need to be fit-tested for an N95 respirator?

Yes. Fit-testing of N95 respirators is required by the Occupational Safety and Health Administration (OSHA) respiratory protection standard (29 CFR 1910.134) when workers could be exposed to hazardous particles or vapors and engineering controls are not feasible (e.g., cleaning up a spill), but often pharmacy personnel are inadvertently excluded from that procedure. Contact your employee health office to let them know that receiving and pharmacy personnel and nursing personnel who handle HDs need to be included in the organization's N95 fit-testing.

8.7-13 My employer has never offered fit-testing of respirators. Can pharmacy staff fit-test each other?

There are specific OSHA requirements that need to be followed. Provision of fit-testing of N95 respirators is required by the OSHA respiratory protection standard (29 CFR 1910.134) when workers could be exposed to hazardous particles or vapors and engineering controls are not feasible (e.g., cleaning up a spill). Information is available at https://www.osha.gov/pls/oshaweb/owadisp.show_document?p_table=STANDARDS&p_id=9780. Be sure your employer is aware of this requirement.

8.7-14 Where can I find information about fit-testing of respirators?

OSHA provides information at https://www.osha.gov/video/respiratory_protection/fittesting_transcript.html.

8.7-15 Does each person handling HDs need his or her own N95 respirator?

You don't necessarily need a separate N95 respirator for each person, but you do need to have available the proper sizes in the proper quantity.

8.7-16 Do I need respiratory protection when I'm cleaning up a spill?

Yes. Respiratory protection is required when cleaning up a spill.

RECEIVING PERSONNEL: HAZARDOUS DRUG PRECAUTIONS 9

(See Sections 5 and 10 in USP <800>.)

APIs of any type of HD and antineoplastic agents must be received using the containment strategies and work practices defined in <800>. <800> allows the entity to perform an Assessment of Risk to evaluate exempting specific dosage forms of HDs from the containment strategies and/or work practices. Non-antineoplastic agents and reproductive hazards may be considered for the entity's Assessment of Risk if alternative containment strategies and/or work practices are identified and implemented.

9.1 What training is required for receiving personnel?

Occupational Safety and Health Administration (OSHA) Hazard Communication Standards and <800> require personnel who handle hazards to be knowledgeable about the risks. Although receiving personnel may not be involved in compounding or administering hazardous drugs (HDs), they need to be aware of occupational risks. The entity's policies need to define the expectations of receiving functions concerning HDs, and they should include the following for receiving personnel:

- Identifying HDs, organizational policies and procedures.
- Use of personal protective equipment (PPE).
- Use of engineering controls and other devices.
- Response to exposure to HDs, spill management, and proper disposal of HDs.

Personnel must document competency prior to independently handling HDs. Personnel training must occur before a new HD or new equipment is used, and competency must be documented at least every 12 months.

9.2 Why is delivery and acceptance of HDs covered under <800>?

The purpose of <800> is to minimize the occupational risk of handling HDs to healthcare personnel. The scope of <800> is wider than in <795> or <797>. <800> is intended to protect healthcare personnel from the time a HD arrives at the organization.

9.3 Where do I open the HDs I receive from suppliers?

If you have a designated negative pressure area for receipt of HDs, open them there. If not, you can open the totes and other packages in your normal receiving area. <800> allows the receiving area to be either negative or neutral/normal pressure. You ***cannot*** receive HDs in a positive pressure area; that would spread contamination if it is present.

9.4 How do I know if a container includes a HD?

Ideally, your supplier will mark the outside of the container with an indication that a HD is inside. This will probably be limited to antineoplastic HDs, as those are the agents that all entities—even those who have performed an Assessment of Risk to exempt some dosage forms of non-antineoplastics or reproductive hazards—will need to handle as HDs.

9.5 Are suppliers required to label HD containers?

<800> does not have the scope to require suppliers to label the containers. However, you can choose to request this from your supplier.

9.6 Do I need a designated room for unpacking? Does it have to be negative?

<800> does not require a designated room, although having a dedicated space to do this is a safe practice that you may want to implement. The space does not have to be negative, but it can be. It *cannot* be positive pressure because that would spread contamination if it is present.

9.7 Should I unpack the wholesaler tote in the chemo room?

No. Do not take the tote or any other outside shipping container into the containment secondary engineering control (C-SEC) (room). These containers have been in dirty environments; you do not want to bring any containers with potential microbial contamination into your International Standards Organization (ISO)-classified areas or into the containment segregated compounding area (C-SCA). Corrugated cardboard can contain mold spores, so you don't want to expose your anteroom or buffer room to that potential contamination. However, if your supplier provides the HDs contained in plastic (e.g., inside a chemo bag) inside your tote, you can remove the plastic bag of HDs and take that bag containing HDs into your negative pressure cleanroom suite or C-SCA.

9.8 Won't I contaminate my C-SEC if I take the wrapped HDs into it?

A compliant C-SEC (room) is designed with negative pressure, external venting, and frequent air changes. This serves to sweep away any particles or contamination.

9.9 Could we use a powder hood to open the packages?

Yes. A containment ventilated enclosure (CVE)—commonly called a powder hood—or a Class I biological safety cabinet (BSC) or other containment primary engineering control (C-PEC) dedicated to receiving and opening HDs would be an ideal situation. This provides a negative pressure device to sweep away the particles.

9.10 What regulations do manufacturers have to control the hazardous residue on the outside of their products?

There are no requirements for suppliers or manufacturers to do this, and requiring it is beyond the scope of <800>. It certainly would improve the safety.

9.11 Do HD totes have to be delivered to the chemo room?

No, and you don't want that to occur. Outside shipping containers or any corrugated cardboard should never be taken into the ISO-classified areas or C-SCAs.

9.12 Would the individual taking the plastic-wrapped package into the buffer room have to be garbed?

Yes. Anyone going into the buffer room needs to be garbed.

9.13 How should the packages of HDs be taken into the chemo room?

Ideally, your supplier wraps the HDs in impervious plastic (e.g., a chemo bag) inside the shipping container. You can take that plastic-wrapped package to the anteroom for receipt by properly garbed compounding personnel. If you have a cleanroom pass-through chamber that goes from the pharmacy into either the anteroom or buffer room, you can take the plastic-wrapped package to that point. If you don't have a pass-through chamber, you could designate cleanable containers (e.g., a tackle box) in which to place the HDs for transport to the anteroom.

9.14 Is there a requirement for pressure monitoring in the receiving area to demonstrate neutral or negative air?

<800> does not require pressure monitoring of the receiving area.

9.15 How should I handle receipt of antineoplastics that will be dispensed without manipulation (e.g., unit-of-use methotrexate tablets)?

This should be evaluated in your Assessment of Risk and a policy developed and in-serviced to staff.

Because packages of oral and topical antineoplastics have the same risk of contamination by HD residue and injections, you might consider these options:

- If you have a designated negative pressure storage area for those antineoplastics that are used for nonsterile compounding, you could take the packages directly to that area.
- If you don't have an area for nonsterile HD compounding, consider keeping them with the injectable antineoplastics that have been received and take all of them into the negative pressure cleanroom. After the compounding staff members have wiped off the containers, use a designated cleanable transport box (e.g., a small tackle box) to move those agents out of the negative pressure cleanroom to the area where they will be stored.
- If you don't have an area for nonsterile HDs and need to package the oral HD into unit-dose or unit-of use containers, consider keeping the unopened bottle in the negative pressure storage area until you first need it. At that point, package the entire bottle using the alternative containment strategies you identify in your Assessment of Risk. After packaging and containment of the entire bottle, you may be able to move the packaged stock into your general storage area if your Assessment of Risk allows.

9.16 What PPE should be available to receiving personnel?

Your policy and procedure need to define what PPE is required for receiving personnel. Chemotherapy gloves tested to American Society for Testing and Materials (ASTM) standard D6978 must be required. The National Institute for Occupational Safety and Health (NIOSH) list of HDs[7] includes a table of suggested PPE for receiving.

<800> requires use of chemotherapy gloves when unpacking HDs. Many personnel in receiving areas wear work gloves; if work gloves are worn, they should be worn over the chemotherapy gloves. If the items received are not enclosed in plastic, <800> recommends wearing an elastomeric half-mask with a multi-gas cartridge and P100 filter until the packaging can be checked to be sure it is not damaged. Protective gowns and respiratory protection are needed if spills or leaks occur, and a spill kit must be available in the receiving area.

9.17 Do I need to wash my hands after I remove the chemo gloves I wear when receiving and stocking chemo agents?

Yes. You need to wash your hands with soap and water any time you remove (doff) any PPE worn when handling HDs. Use of alcohol hand rub alone is *not* sufficient.

9.18 How should damaged or broken HD containers be handled?

The entity needs to have a policy and procedure in place for this situation, and receiving personnel must have documented competency. A stratified approach is needed. See **Table 9-1** for policy requirements and recommendations.

9.19 What happens if a damaged package needs to be opened?

The entity must have a policy and procedure in place for this situation, and receiving personnel need to have documented competency. A stratified approach is necessary. See Table 9-1 for policy requirements and recommendations.

9.20 We segregate antineoplastic deliveries from our wholesaler by using a unique PO number. Do non-antineoplastics (e.g., warfarin, estrogen, fluconazole) need to be in separate totes?

It depends on your Assessment of Risk. If you have identified alternative containment strategies (e.g., purchasing manufacturer unit dose, premixed infusions), you may choose to handle the non-antineoplastic agents and reproductive hazards that are in final dosage forms the same way as you handle non-HDs. If you use a process to separate antineoplastics from other agents by using a separate purchase order (PO) number, you could use the same process to separate out the other HDs.

9.21 Will wholesalers designate hazardous items in their ordering system?

That is up to the wholesaler or other supplier. There is no requirement to do this in <800>, since that is out of scope of <800>.

9.22 Do I have to receive HDs in a negative pressure area?

No. The HDs can be received in either a neutral/normal pressure area or in a negative pressure area. No corrugated cardboard or external shipping containers should be brought into a negative pressure area.

TABLE 9-1 Requirements and Recommendations for Receiving Hazardous Drugs

Observe Contents of Package	Minimum PPE Required	Receiving Area	Recommended Procedure
All intact and enclosed in impervious plastic bag	1 pair chemotherapy gloves	Can be received in neutral/normal, or negative pressure, but the negative pressure area cannot be the sterile compounding negative pressure room. DO NOT receive this in a positive pressure area.	Remove bag of HDs from the external container, then take the unopened bag to be placed in the negative pressure storage area
All intact but not enclosed in an impervious plastic bag	2 pairs chemotherapy gloves, impervious gown, shoe covers, respiratory protection	Ideally, in a separate negative pressure area. Neutral/normal pressure area is acceptable. DO NOT receive this in a positive pressure area.	Contain the HD by placing it in plastic or another impervious container, then place the container in the negative pressure storage area
Damaged and will not be opened	2 pairs chemotherapy gloves, impervious gown, shoe covers, respiratory protection		Seal the container and contact the supplier. Ideally, the supplier will provide credit and tell you to discard the package as hazardous waste. If the package must be returned to the supplier, enclose it in an impervious container and label the outer container as hazardous. Segregate HDs waiting to be returned to the supplier in a designated negative pressure area. Report the damaged package as a spill, using your organization's procedure for reporting spills.
Damaged but need to open the package to retrieve one or more undamaged product	2 pairs chemotherapy gloves, impervious gown, shoe covers, respiratory protection		Seal the container in plastic or in an impervious container. Take it to a C-PEC (preferably one used only for nonsterile preparations), open the package on a disposable plastic mat, and remove the undamaged items. Wipe the outside of the undamaged items with a disposable wipe. Place the undamaged items in the negative pressure storage area. Decontaminate and clean the C-PEC. Discard the wipes and mat as hazardous waste. Ideally, the supplier will provide credit for the damaged items and tell you to discard the package as hazardous waste. If the package must be returned to the supplier, enclose it in an impervious container and label the outer container as hazardous. Segregate HDs waiting to be returned to the supplier in a designated negative pressure area. Report the damaged package as a spill, using your organization's procedure for reporting spills.

C-PEC: containment primary engineering control; HD: hazardous drug; HDs: hazardous drugs; PPE: personal protective equipment

9.23 How can I identify HD containers when they come in from suppliers?

Your supplier should identify the outside of the container if antineoplastic agents are included in a package. Ideally, only antineoplastics will be in a tote or other container separate from other drugs. Some pharmacies separate their supplier orders so only antineoplastics are ordered on a single PO; that generally forces the supplier to package them separately.

9.24 How should HDs be packaged by suppliers?

Because most organizations are expected to use an Assessment of Risk approach, only the antineoplastic agents are likely to be segregated. Your supplier should identify the container by a different color tote or a distinctive label on the outside of the container and should wrap the antineoplastic agents inside the marked container in impervious plastic.

9.25 Where should HD shipments be received?

HD containers should be delivered to the area where they will be used. In most pharmacies, this means to the general pharmacy receiving area (not a loading dock). The HDs have to be delivered to the HD storage area immediately after they are received and unpacked.

9.26 What garb needs to be worn by receiving personnel?

At least one pair of chemotherapy gloves must be worn when receiving HDs. Facility policy may require other PPE for routine use and must require additional PPE if HDs are received not in impervious plastic or are damaged. The receiving area must have a spill kit.

9.27 What is the ideal process for receiving HDs?

Ideally, all totes and other containers arrive with an identifiable marking, indicating that antineoplastic HDs—and only antineoplastic HDs—are inside. The properly garbed receiving person opens the container and finds the antineoplastic HDs wrapped in a sealed, impervious plastic wrap. The drugs are visible through the plastic, so the receiving list can be checked without opening the sealed plastic bag. Once the contents are reconciled, the sealed plastic bag is transported into the negative pressure buffer room or C-SCA through a pass-through that meets <797> and <800> criteria. The bag of antineoplastic HDs is then opened in the negative pressure storage room, the negative pressure buffer room, or C-SCA and placed in stock in plastic bins in that room.

9.28 Should receiving personnel open up all the boxes of chemotherapy?

External shipping containers and any corrugated cardboard should be removed by receiving personnel. Smooth coated cardboard boxes in which many antineoplastic vials are packaged can remain unopened. Smooth, coated cardboard packaging is acceptable to be placed in the negative pressure area as long as the negative pressure area can maintain the required controls (e.g., ISO classification).

9.29 What should be done when broken or damaged HDs are received?

The entity must have a policy and procedure in place for this situation, and receiving personnel need to have competency documented concerning it. A stratified approach is necessary. See Table 9-1 for policy requirements and recommendations.

STORAGE OF HAZARDOUS DRUGS 10

(See Section 5 in USP <800>.)

APIs of any type of HD and antineoplastic agents (with the potential entity-exemption of antineoplastics that need to be only counted or packaged) must be stored using the containment strategies and work practices defined in <800>. An entity's Assessment of Risk may exempt specific dosage forms of those agents listed in the NIOSH HD list tables for non-antineoplastics and reproductive hazards or those antineoplastics that need to be only counted or packaged if alternative containment strategies and/or work practices are identified and implemented.

10.1 What are the minimum storage requirements for the location of HD storage?

Hazardous drugs (HDs) must be stored in a room with fixed walls (not plastic curtains) that is separate from non-HD storage. The room must have a negative pressure between 0.01 to 0.03" wc, be vented to the outside, and have at least 12 air changes per hour (ACPH).

10.2 Am I required to store all HDs in a negative pressure room?

You must store any active pharmaceutical ingredients (APIs) of any HD in a negative pressure room. You must store any antineoplastic HD that has to be manipulated in a negative pressure room. The other agents and dosage forms are based on your Assessment of Risk. If you don't do an Assessment of Risk, all must be stored in a negative pressure room.

<800> allows you to perform an Assessment of Risk for
- antineoplastic agents that need to be only counted or packaged;
- non-antineoplastic agents; and
- reproductive hazards.

If your Assessment of Risk permits, you may not have to store those agents in a negative pressure room, but you have to identify how you mitigate the risks to personnel by identifying alternative containment strategies.

10.3 Where does <800> say that I have to keep two sets of inventory—one for nonsterile and one for sterile?

There is no requirement in <800> for two sets of inventory. You need to keep all HDs (unless entity-exempted in your Assessment of Risk) in negative pressure.

10.4 Are manufacturers required to clean the outer packaging of unit-dose/unit-of-use containers?

No, that is one of the reasons why HDs must be stored in negative pressure and separated from non-hazardous agents.

10.5 Why do HDs need to be stored in a negative room?

The negative room is used to contain the hazardous residue that may be on the outside of packages. There is no requirement by the U.S. Food and Drug Administration (FDA) or other regulators to ship packages that are free of HD residue. Because drugs need to be moved from storage to the compounding area, using a negative pressure storage area protects adjacent areas from the contamination.

10.6 Can I store HDs in the negative pressure buffer room?

Yes, you can store HDs in the negative pressure buffer room since the room exceeds the minimum requirements for storage as long as (1) you have adequate room for the storage and (2) the room maintains the required standards for certification. However, you cannot store any external containers (e.g., shipping containers, wholesaler totes) or corrugated cardboard in that area because it would introduce the potential for microbial contamination. You should store items intended only for sterile compounding in a negative pressure buffer room intended for sterile HD compounding.

10.7 Can HD and non-HD APIs be stored in the same negative pressure room if they are separated?

It depends what you do with your non-HD APIs. Is it used only for HD compounding? In that case, it could be acceptable. But if it's used for non-HD compounding, you would have to label any preparation with personal protective equipment (PPE) precautions. That is likely not an acceptable or practical way to handle this.

10.8 Do all my non-chemo agents need to be in a negative room?

All antineoplastic agents (with the potential exception of those final dosage forms that need to be only counted and/or packaged) and all APIs have to be in a negative pressure storage room. Storage of the non-antineoplastics and reproductive hazards on the National Institute for Occupational Safety and Health (NIOSH) list of HDs may not need to be stored in a negative pressure room if you conduct an Assessment of Risk and define alternative containment strategies and/or work practices.

10.9 If I use an injection for nonsterile compounding, where do I store it?

If it could be used for either nonsterile or sterile compounding, store it in the sterile compounding negative storage area, and develop a procedure to outline how it will be removed from that area and by whom. If it is used only for nonsterile compounding, it could be stored in the nonsterile compounding negative storage area.

10.10 What does *antineoplastic requiring only counting or packaging* mean?

You may handle some antineoplastics such as methotrexate tablets in unit-of-use containers or conventionally manufactured fluorouracil cream that you do not manipulate. If you identify alternative containment strategies in your Assessment of Risk, they could be stored with your other stock rather than in a negative pressure storage area. If you handle some antineoplastic solid oral forms that do not produce powder or vapors, you might be able to identify alternative containment strategies in your Assessment of Risk to allow those agents to be stored with your other stock rather than in a negative pressure storage area.

10.11 Do I have to post a sign at the front door of the pharmacy stating that HDs are stored inside?

No, unless state or other regulations require it. Post the sign on the door(s) to the HD storage and compounding areas.

10.12 Do oral HDs have to be stored in a negative pressure room?

If you identify alternative containment strategies in your Assessment of Risk, they could be stored with your other stock in neutral/normal pressure rather than in a negative pressure storage area. If you handle some antineoplastic solid oral forms that do not produce powder or vapors, you might be able to identify alternative containment strategies in your Assessment of Risk to allow those agents to be stored with your other stock rather than in a negative pressure storage area.

10.13 What examples of alternative containment strategies could we consider for oral antineoplastic agents to allow them to be stored with regular stock?

Consider a process such as wiping down the packaging when received, storing them in lidded yellow plastic bins, and using a separate counting tray and spatula that would be decontaminated after use.

10.14 Can I store chemo with other stock?

Injectable antineoplastics (unless only counted or packaged) must be stored in a negative pressure storage room. Antineoplastics that need to be only counted or packaged may be stored with other stock if you have identified alternative containment strategies in your Assessment of Risk.

10.15 Can hazardous and chemotherapy drugs be stored in the same area?

If you are asking whether antineoplastic agents can be stored in the same area as other HDs on the NIOSH list, it depends if you perform an Assessment of Risk. You must store the antineoplastic agents separately from non-HDs. If you don't perform an Assessment of Risk, or if your assessment of risk determines that you will store some or all of the non-antineoplastic and/or reproductive hazards as you would antineoplastic agents, then yes—you could store them together. However, you then need to treat all of those drugs as you would chemo agents because they could be contaminated with HD residue. More likely, you will want to perform an Assessment of Risk for the non-antineoplastics and reproductive hazards and store them with alternative containment strategies.

10.16 Can I store all my drugs (i.e., hazardous and non-hazardous) in a single negative pressure room?

That is not a practical approach. The reason for the negative pressure room is to contain any hazardous residue and remove it by proper ventilation. If you stored your non-HDs in that same area, you would potentially contaminate all your drug packages. You would also need to put all non-HDs in a protective bag and label them with PPE precautions.

10.17 Can I store nonsterile chemo drugs in my sterile chemo room?

Think of your work practices. To enter your sterile compounding area, you need to be fully garbed. You don't want unauthorized personnel entering the sterile compounding area. Would storage of nonsterile antineoplastics in the sterile compounding area compromise those principles? In most cases, it would, so you would want to avoid doing this.

However, you might have a practice where unopened bottles of oral antineoplastic agents are stored in your negative pressure buffer area awaiting packaging. If that is your practice, you would need to establish a clear work plan to ensure that only authorized entry occurs and how you will handle the oral agents after they are packaged.

10.18 I don't have room in my negative pressure buffer room to store stock. Can I use a vented flammable cabinet?

A standard flammable cabinet will not meet the requirements for storage (separate room, negative pressure, vented to the outside, and at least 12 ACPH). However, if a cabinet can be purchased that meets those requirements, it could be used for storage. You would also need to develop a work practice to transport the items from that cabinet (which would essentially be the "room") to your compounding area.

10.19 I have a negative pressure room with a negative pressure cabinet that is used to store all of our HD APIs. We keep other items in the cabinet that are not hazardous. Do we need to remove the non-HD items from there?

Are these items used for HD preparations? If that's the case, you may be OK with where they are. Anything in the room is potentially contaminated, so you need to consider that. It's similar to mixing non-HD medications in a biological safety cabinet (BSC); you would have to label it with PPE precautions and put it in a protective bag so it wouldn't contaminate other items. If you are talking about a lot of non-HD medications and supplies, or a non-HD API that's always used for non-HD preparations, it is a different issue and should be moved out of the HD area.

10.20 Where can I obtain a list of hazardous medications that release volatile vapors during storage?

Unfortunately, there isn't a master list of these drugs. This information has come from published articles. One reference titled "Vapour pressures, evaporation behavior and airborne concentrations of hazardous drugs: implications for occupational safety" is available at https://www.researchgate.net/profile/Thekla_Kiffmeyer/publication/240640598_Vapour_pressures_evaporation_behaviour_and_airborne_concentrations_of_hazardous_drugs_Implications_for_occupational_safety/links/5436559c0cf2643ab986c5ac.pdf.

10.21 Does USP <797> allow storage in the buffer area?

There is no restriction for storage in USP <797>. The test is whether the room meets International Standards Organization (ISO) 7 requirements during use. As long as the room will meet the ISO 7 requirements under dynamic (working) conditions and you have the room for storage, you may store the HD items in the negative pressure buffer room. However, never bring in any external shipping containers or corrugated cardboard into the sterile compounding area. The smooth-coated cardboard in which many antineoplastic agents are packaged is generally not a problem.

10.22 Where do I store HDs that require refrigeration?

Refrigerated antineoplastic agents must be stored in a dedicated refrigerator in your negative pressure storage area. If you have identified alternative containment strategies in your Assessment of Risk for dosage forms of HDs that aren't antineoplastics, you may be able to store those agents in your refrigerator with non-hazardous stock.

10.23 What are my options for storing refrigerated HDs?

For those drugs that are APIs and those that are antineoplastics (unless they are final dosage forms that need to be only counted or packaged), you must keep them in a refrigerator dedicated to HD (only) storage in your negative pressure room.

See Section 14, Design of Compounding Facilities, for more information about refrigerator placement.

If you have performed an Assessment of Risk and determined alternative containment strategies and/or work practices for HDs that are not APIs or not antineoplastic, you can store those non-antineoplastic and reproductive HDs with your other drugs. In most cases, it may mean that you identify them as hazards but store them in the same refrigerator you use for storage of non-HDs.

10.24 Does the refrigerator have to be a negative pressure refrigerator?

No, but the refrigerator needs to be in a negative pressure room.

10.25 I have only one pharmacy refrigerator. Can I designate one shelf to store antineoplastics?

If you will be manipulating those antineoplastics (e.g., for compounding), then *no*; you need a separate refrigerator for those agents, and it must be in your negative pressure room. If you have only antineoplastics that you will only count or package, you may store them in your regular pharmacy refrigerator if you have identified alternative containment strategies for those specific dosage forms in your Assessment of Risk.

10.26 Can I store chemo vials in smooth-coated cardboard boxes in my negative pressure buffer room?

Yes, as long as you have adequate room to do that and as long as the room meets the certification requirements.

10.27 Can I store saline vials and other similar non-hazardous items in the negative pressure buffer room?

Yes, as long as you have adequate room to do that and as long as the room meets the certification requirements. Once you have exposed non-hazardous adjunct medications (e.g., saline vials) in the negative pressure storage room, anteroom, buffer room, or containment segregated compounding area (C-SCA), you must consider them like HDs. You could not then use them for non-hazardous compounds or dispensing.

10.28 Would it be reasonable to store a limited number of oncology support (e.g., anti-emetics) medication to be stored alongside HD in a C-SCA where the compounding takes place? It sounds like this is prohibited.

That is acceptable. You would just need to restrict those agents for HD compounding and label them as such. You could not then use them for non-hazardous compounds or dispensing.

10.29 Can I use a flammable cabinet to store my chemo?

No, you cannot use a flammable cabinet to store chemo unless the cabinet is vented to the outside, has the required negative pressure, and has at least 12 ACPH. General flammable cabinets do not meet these criteria.

10.30 Can HDs be stored in a negative pressure cabinet located in a neutral area?

No, this would not meet the required containment. Consider what would occur if an item falls and breaks when it is being removed from the cabinet; it would contaminate the entire area.

10.31 Do I understand correctly that not only do chemo agents need to be compounded in a negative pressure room, but they also need to be stored there prior to use even if they are in a manufacturer's sealed box?

Yes, antineoplastic agents that will be manipulated in any way need to be both stored and compounded in a negative room. This doesn't have to be the same room. Exposure to HDs isn't limited to compounding; the outside of the manufacturer's box could be contaminated or the box could fall and break prior to compounding.

10.32 Would the separation of HDs and non-HDs include storage of large quantities in original packaging prior to unpacking for prescription packaging?

Large quantities of HDs intended for packaging should be stored with the containment strategies listed in <800>. Although technically you could use the allowance for dosage forms intended only for counting and packaging, consider the volume of hazard you are manipulating.

10.33 What are the recommendations regarding refrigerator placement for refrigerated antineoplastic HDs? USP <797> allows placement in a negative pressure buffer room; however, <800> recommendations indicate exhaust placement near the compressor and behind unit.

These are not different requirements; <800> provides more guidance in placement of the refrigerator. Your refrigerator—or any device that could produce particles—should be placed near an exhaust to allow the particles generated to be swept out of the room.

10.34 Can hazardous and chemotherapy drugs be stored in the same area?

If you are asking whether antineoplastic agents can be stored in the same area as other HDs on the NIOSH list, it depends if you perform an Assessment of Risk. You must store the antineoplastic agents separately from non-HDs. If you don't perform an Assessment of Risk, or if your Assessment of Risk determines that you will store some or all of the non-antineoplastic and/or reproductive hazards as you would antineoplastic agents, then yes—you could store them together. However, you then need to treat all of those drugs as you would chemo agents because they could be contaminated with HD residue. More likely, you will want to perform an Assessment of Risk for the non-antineoplastics and reproductive hazards and store them with alternative containment strategies.

10.35 Is it acceptable to store HDs in automated dispensing cabinets?

Consider this in your Assessment of Risk. For any antineoplastics, consider the risk of contamination of the entire automated dispensing cabinet (ADC) if a breakage occurs. You would need to remove the ADC from service if that occurred. However, specific dosage forms of non-antineoplastics or reproductive hazards may not all have the same risk.

10.36 Is it acceptable to store HDs in carousels?

Consider this in your Assessment of Risk. For any antineoplastics, consider the risk of contamination of the entire carousel if a breakage occurs. You would need to remove the carousel from service if that occurred. However, specific dosage forms of non-antineoplastics or reproductive hazards may not have the same risk.

10.37 If the material is not volatile, why must negative pressure storage be used?

Some antineoplastic drugs volatilize at room temperature. Studies have demonstrated that antineoplastic vial packages are contaminated with HD residue. Stock can fall from shelving and break. Negative pressure rooms that are vented to the outside and have at least 12 ACPH protect the contamination from any of these situations from reaching adjacent areas.

10.38 What are the storage area requirements for a nursing unit?

Only final or finished dosage forms should be dispensed to patient care or procedural areas. Your Assessment of Risk should identify the designated storage area. Antineoplastics should be dispensed in impervious containers (e.g., chemo bags) so the potential for contamination is mitigated. There is no requirement for negative storage for patient care or procedural areas handling only final or finished dosage forms that are properly contained.

10.39 Can intact (unopened) HDs be stored in neutral/normal pressure areas in addition to negative pressure rooms?

APIs of any HD or any antineoplastic agents that require manipulation need to be stored in a negative pressure room. These drugs can be received in neutral/normal pressure areas but should be moved to a negative pressure storage area as soon as possible. Your Assessment of Risk may identify specific dosage forms of HDs that are non-antineoplastics or reproductive hazards that could be stored in neutral/normal pressure areas.

10.40 We were compliant with <797> storage; it said "separate." Why does this now need to be negative?

<800> provides more detailed definitions of handling HDs than <797> did. <800> is intended to protect healthcare personnel from occupational risks associated with handling HDs, and negative pressure storage is one element of it.

10.41 How do you transport inventory that has been received into a negative pressure room?

If you have a cleanroom-compliant pass-through between your receiving area and your negative pressure room, you can use it. Ideally, your HDs are received in an impervious plastic bag (e.g., chemo bag) that can be transported (without opening it) through your pass-through into the negative pressure room.

If you don't have a pass-through, your Assessment of Risk needs to identify the containment strategies you will use to protect personnel and non-negative areas from contamination.

You might consider use of a designated tackle box to minimize the chance of packaged breaking or leaking. The tackle box could be lined with a plastic-backed pad, and the box would need to be decontaminated after use.

10.42 Can I use a pneumatic tube to transport chemo items to our satellite pharmacy?

Pneumatic tube systems **cannot** be used to transport any antineoplastic agent or liquid forms of any HD due to the potential to contaminate the entire tube system if the HD leaks or breaks.

10.43 The only injectable antineoplastic we stock is methotrexate for ectopic pregnancy. How should this be stored?

It needs to be stored in a negative pressure room. It also needs to be prepared in a containment primary engineering control (C-PEC) in a negative pressure anteroom/buffer room suite or in a C-SCA. *It is not appropriate—nor compliant with <800>—to simply send the vial to a patient care unit for nursing to draw up.*

10.44 <797> states that drugs are not to be stored in the buffer area or anteroom, so why does <800> allow for storage of drugs and refrigerators in the buffer room?

There is no such restriction in <797>. The test of an anteroom and buffer room is the ability to meet the certification standards. Of course, this needs to be reasonable. It would be inappropriate to use your anteroom or buffer room for large quantities of drug storage.

10.45 Does storage in a negative pressure room include both oral and injectable medications?

If you have a negative pressure room dedicated for storage, you could store all dosage forms of HDs in it. Most facilities do not have a separate negative storage area, so they use the negative pressure sterile buffer room for storage of injectable antineoplastics. HDs used for nonsterile compounding should not be stored in the sterile compounding area to minimize traffic into the sterile compounding space.

10.46 My workplace is a community pharmacy. Do I need a separate room for all HDs or just for the antineoplastics?

If you are dealing only with final dosage forms that you only count or package, you may not need a separate room if you perform an Assessment of Risk and determine that no other manipulation is occurring.

10.47 Does the area where I place HDs awaiting return to suppliers have to be separate from the regular HD storage area?

A separate room is not required, but the items awaiting return need to be segregated in a designated space within the negative pressure storage room.

COUNTING AND PACKAGING HAZARDOUS DRUGS

(See Sections 2 and 12 in USP <800>.)

<800> allows the entity to perform an Assessment of Risk to evaluate exempting specific dosage forms of HDs from the containment strategies and/or work practices. Antineoplastics that require only counting or packaging can be considered in the Assessment of Risk.

11.1 Can I continue to package non-antineoplastics and reproductive hazards using automated packaging machines?

Consider this in your Assessment of Risk. In most cases, you may be comfortable continuing your current practices for those agents that are non-antineoplastics or reproductive hazards. However, assess if those agents volatilize and/or produce powders as these are risks to personnel. You may want to restrict certain dosage forms of these agents to a manual packaging system.

11.2 How should I package unit-dose solid oral antineoplastics?

Use only a manual packaging method for antineoplastics. Do not use an automated counting or packaging system because tablets or capsules that break would contaminate the equipment. Consider packaging antineoplastics in a containment primary engineering control (C-PEC) in a negative pressure buffer room or containment segregated compounding area (C-SCA). Ideally, this would be done in a C-PEC used for nonsterile compounding, but if the only C-PEC available is used for sterile compounding, the packaging would need to be done while no sterile compounding was occurring. The C-PEC must be decontaminated, cleaned, and disinfected prior to re-use for sterile compounding.

11.3 If I buy only manufacturer unit-dose or unit-of-use packages, can I store the HDs—even antineoplastics—with my regular stock?

Evaluate this in your Assessment of Risk. <800> allows the entity to exempt certain dosage forms from negative pressure storage. If you do store antineoplastics with regular stock, consider some type of alternative containment (e.g., lidded plastic storage bins).

11.4 What would be an example of how a pharmacy could package unit-dose oral antineoplastic agents and be compliant with USP <800>?

One approach might be to package the entire bottle of tablets at one time. For example, unit-dose bubble-pack the entire bottle of tablets in the biological safety cabinet (BSC), using the full personal protective equipment (PPE) that you would for compounding. Label it to meet your policies. Place the unit doses into a designated bin. Because you have taken several levels of precautions, you might (if your Assessment of Risk allows) store these in your general storage area.

What would be an example of how a community pharmacy should count out oral antineoplastic agents?

One approach might be to dedicate a specific counting tray and spatula for antineoplastic agents. One pair of chemotherapy gloves tested to American Society for Testing and Materials (ASTM) D6978 should be worn while handling the antineoplastic agent. Decontaminate and clean the counting tray and spatula after each use.

See Section 21, Decontamination and Cleaning, for further information.

TYPES OF ENGINEERING CONTROLS 12

(See <800> Section 5, Appendix 2, and Appendix 3 in USP <800>.)

Engineering controls are used to contain hazards. <800> describes three types of engineering controls: *primary* (the hood), *secondary* (the room in which the primary control is placed), and *supplemental* (closed system drug-transfer devices used for compounding and administration). If alternative containment strategies and/or work practices are defined in the Assessment of Risk, the entity may exempt specific dosage forms of non-antineoplastic agents and reproductive hazards and dosage forms of antineoplastics that are only counted or packaged from some engineering control requirements.

12.1 GENERAL INFORMATION

12.1-1 What are the types of engineering controls?

Three types of engineering controls are defined in <800>:

1. *Containment primary engineering control* (C-PEC)—the device in which compounds are mixed, including a containment ventilated enclosure (CVE) commonly called *powder hoods*, a biological safety cabinet (BSC), and a compounding aseptic containment isolator (CACI).
2. *Containment secondary engineering control* (C-SEC)—the room in which the C-PEC is placed, including the anteroom/buffer room suite or a containment segregated compounding area (C-SCA).
3. *Supplemental engineering controls*—closed system drug-transfer devices (CSTDs), which are devices that mechanically prohibit the transfer of environmental contaminants into the system and the escape of hazardous drug (HD) or vapor concentrations outside the system.

12.1-2 How do the PECs in <800> differ from those in <797>?

The PECs for compounding sterile HDs are the same. <800> also requires PECs for nonsterile HD compounding. The *containment* term is added to designate use with HDs.

12.1-3 How do the SECs in <800> differ from those in <797>?

A cleanroom suite as a SEC has the same structure as in <797>, but <800> adds in some additional requirements. The *containment* term is added to designate use with HDs. (*See Section 14, Design of Compounding Facilities.*) <797> allows placement of a BSC or CACI in a positive pressure room if only a low volume of hazardous compounding is done; <800> does not allow that. <800> allows a C-SCA, which is a new configuration not permitted by <797>.

12.1-4 How do the supplemental engineering controls in <800> differ from those in <797>?

The term *supplemental engineering control* does not appear in <797>, although CSTDs are included. In <797>, CSTDs are required if you have a BSC or CACI in a positive pressure buffer room. In <800>, that configuration is not permitted. In <800>, CSTDs are recommended for use when compounding and required for use during administration of HDs if the dosage form allows.

12.1-5 What is a *C-PEC*?

A *C-PEC* is the hood where the preparations are compounded. USP <800> defines a C-PEC as a "ventilated device designed and operated to minimize worker and environmental exposures to HDs by controlling emissions of airborne contaminants through a full or partial enclosure of a potential contaminant source, the use of airflow capture velocities to trap and remove airborne contaminants near their point of generation, the use of air pressure relationships that define the direction of airflow into the cabinet, and the use of HEPA filtration on all potentially contaminated exhaust streams."[8]

12.1-6 Do certain drugs require use of a CACI instead of a BSC?

No. Either a CACI or a BSC can be used as your PEC; there is no distinction between them based on what drugs you are compounding.

12.1-7 What are the basic requirements for a BSC for sterile compounding?

Only Class II BSCs are appropriate for sterile compounding. Class II BSCs provide worker, preparation, and environmental protection. Be sure to get a BSC that is on the list of NSF Certified Biosafety Cabinetry (http://info.nsf.org/Certified/Biosafety/), which has been independently performance-verified. Standard Class II BSCs that you can purchase will be on this list. If you need a special order BSC for some reason, ask the manufacturer to perform the biological test that they would use for certification of the unit.

12.1-8 What is a *containment ventilated enclosure*?

A *CVE* is a type of C-PEC used for nonsterile compounding, commonly called a *powder hood*.

12.1-9 What additional items should be considered if my CVE will have redundant HEPA filters instead of being vented to the outside?

External venting is preferred; but if you will have a CVE that has redundant high-efficiency particulate air (HEPA) filters, be sure that both filters will be able to be leak tested. If the CVE is used to protect against drugs that volatilize at room temperature, it needs to be externally vented.

12.1-10 What is a *containment secondary engineering control*?

A *C-SEC* is a room with fixed walls in which the C-PEC is placed. The room is under negative pressure, is vented to the outside, and has an appropriate number of air changes per hour (ACPH). Ideally, for sterile compounding, this is a suite of rooms (positive pressure anteroom

12.1-11 What is a *containment segregated compounding area*?

A *C-SCA* is a type of C-SEC with nominal requirements for air flow and room pressurization as they pertain to HD compounding. The room with fixed walls is under negative pressure, is vented to the outside, and has at least 12 ACPH but is not required to meet ISO Class 7 standards.

12.1-12 What is a *supplemental engineering control*?

A *supplemental engineering control* is a "CSTD, which mechanically prohibits the transfer of environmental contaminants into the system and the escape of HD or vapor concentrations outside the system."[8]

12.1-13 Do HEPA filters stop gases?

No. They only trap particles, which is why the compounding space needs to be externally vented. This is what sweeps away the vapors.

12.2 CONTAINMENT PRIMARY ENGINEERING CONTROLS FOR NONSTERILE COMPOUNDING

12.2-1 What is a *primary engineering control*?

The *PEC* is a ventilated device in which you prepare your compounds. It is designed to minimize personnel and environmental HD exposure when compounding HDs.

12.2-2 Does nonsterile HD compounding require a C-PEC?

Nonsterile compounding of active pharmaceutical ingredients (APIs) of any type of HD or of antineoplastics requires a C-PEC. The entity may perform an Assessment of Risk for specific dosage forms of those HDs that are non-antineoplastic or reproductive hazards.

12.2-3 What types of C-PECs are compliant for compounding nonsterile HDs?

Compliant C-PECs for nonsterile hazardous compounding include CVEs (commonly called a *powder hood*), Class I or II BSCs, or a CACI. The C-PEC must protect personnel and the environment.

12.2-4 Does the C-PEC used for nonsterile compounding need to be vented to the outside?

External venting is preferred, but the C-PEC can alternatively have redundant HEPA filters in series if it is not externally vented. The room in which the C-PEC is placed must be externally vented.

12.2-5 What does *redundant HEPA filters in series* mean?

If the C-PEC for nonsterile HD compounding is not externally vented, you need to be sure that there is a backup if one of the HEPA filters fail. Placing an additional HEPA filter in the same line (in series) provides the redundancy for safety.

12.2-6 Can redundant HEPA filters in series be used instead of external venting if volatile agents are compounded?

If volatile agents are compounded, external venting—*not* the alternative for redundant HEPA filters in series—should be employed.

12.2-7 Does the pre-filter count as one of the HEPA filters?

No, the two filters in series must be HEPA filters.

12.2-8 Can the C-PEC for nonsterile compounding be vented into another room instead of to the outside?

No. If it is vented, it must be vented to the outside.

12.2-9 What should I look for when buying a powder hood or CVE?

Until more definitive information is available from the Controlled Environment Testing Association (CETA), the manufacturer should provide documentation that the device meets the standard of the American Society of Heating, Refrigerating, and Air-Conditioning Engineers (ASHRE) 110, which is a performance test for laboratory fume hoods.

12.2-10 I make only two or three nonsterile chemo preparations a year. Can I use my BSC in the sterile compounding room to do this?

Yes. <800> allows use of the sterile compounding C-PEC and room for occasional nonsterile compounding, *provided you comply with certain restrictions:* no sterile compounding can be done while you are using the room for nonsterile compounding and the C-PEC must be decontaminated, cleaned, and disinfected prior to using the room for sterile compounding.

12.2-11 What is *occasional* nonsterile compounding? At what point do I need a separate hood?

There is no number defined in <800>. Consider this as part of your Assessment of Risk. If you do this every day, or even every week, it's not occasional. If it's your business plan to provide HD nonsterile compounds, it's not occasional. You need the proper equipment for the compounds you mix.

12.2-12 How should community pharmacies that dispense a large number of the drugs on the NIOSH list handle <800>?

If you handle API of any of the HDs on the National Institute for Occupational Safety and Health (NIOSH) list or manipulate any antineoplastics (other than counting and packaging them), you need to comply with all the containment strategies and work practices listed in

<800>. If you handle only the non-antineoplastics and reproductive hazards and only count or package final dosage forms of antineoplastics, you may perform an Assessment of Risk to define alternative containment strategies and/or work practices.

12.2-13 The only antineoplastic agent I stock is methotrexate tablets. I need to count out tablets, and sometimes there is powder in the container. How does <800> deal with that situation?

<800> allows the entity to perform an Assessment of Risk concerning this situation. Could the tablets be purchased in a unit-of-use container? That way, you would not need to expose personnel to the powder. If this is a common occurrence, you might want to consider use of a powder hood to count and package the drug. If this is an unusual situation, you could include in your Assessment of Risk an approach similar to receiving damaged packages (see Table 9-1).

12.2-14 The only risk I have is to package unit-dose methotrexate tabs. I don't have a BSC. Can I turn off my regular laminar air flow positive pressure hood and package them there?

No. A laminar air flow hood used for preparation of non-hazardous mixtures is positive pressure. You cannot use a positive pressure PEC for manipulation of HDs. Even by turning off the hood (which should never be done except for servicing or moving it), you would be contaminating that surface. <800> allows counting and packaging oral antineoplastic agents if alternative containment strategies are identified in your Assessment of Risk, but turning off your positive pressure PEC is not an acceptable method of containment.

12.2-15 How should we prepare single doses of HDs when we need to make an oral liquid from a tablet or capsule?

If the agent is an antineoplastic, you need to do that in a C-PEC in a C-SEC. If the agent is a HD that is non-antineoplastic or a reproductive hazard, you may determine entity exemptions for specific dosage forms in your Assessment of Risk if you define and implement alternative containment strategies and/or work practices.

12.2-16 We currently use a non-externally vented CACI for preparation of oral HDs (i.e., drawing up pediatric liquid oral HD, compounding extemporaneous HD liquids from tablets). Per <800>, will this still be acceptable or will it need to be externally vented?

If this is used exclusively for nonsterile compounding, there are two options. Ideally, it should be externally vented, but <800> also allows PECs used only for nonsterile compounding to have redundant HEPA filters in series if the device is not vented. However, if it is also used for sterile compounding, it must be externally vented.

12.2-17 Can nonsterile compounds be prepared in a negative pressure room in a BSC?

Yes, either a Class I or II BSC can be used. Other acceptable PECs for nonsterile compounding are CVEs (commonly called *powder hoods*) or CACIs.

12.2-18 It is my understanding that when USP <800> goes into effect that all chemicals considered hazardous need to be stored in a separate room, which contains a positive pressure powder hood vented to the outside and for which all compounding must be performed. Is this correct?

No. <800> deals with those drugs on the NIOSH list of HDs. It does not deal with other chemicals or drugs considered hazardous by the Environmental Protection Agency (EPA) or other organizations. There is no requirement in <800> for a positive pressure powder hood because that would be counter to the containment properties you want to use for HDs.

12.2-19 Does the powder hood need to have a filtration system in addition to venting outside or does venting out suffice?

The C-PEC used for nonsterile compounding (often called a *powder hood*) can either be externally vented or can have redundant HEPA filters in series. If it is vented outside—which is preferred—there is no requirement for it to also have HEPA filters in the vent as long as there is a HEPA filter in the powder hood.

12.2-20 Is there an industry guidance for testing/certification of a powder hood?

Until more definitive information is available from CETA, ask your certifier to use the ASHRE 110 test to check if the device works properly and is integrated into the facility.

12.3 CONTAINMENT PRIMARY ENGINEERING CONTROLS FOR STERILE COMPOUNDING

12.3-1 What is a *primary engineering control*?

A *C-PEC* is the ventilated device in which you prepare your compounds. It is designed to minimize personnel and environmental HD exposure when compounding HDs.

12.3-2 What types of C-PECs are compliant for compounding sterile HDs?

Compliant C-PECs for sterile hazardous compounding include Class II BSCs and CACIs. There are also some robotic devices that meet the requirements of a CACI. The C-PEC used for sterile HD compounding must protect personnel and the environment as well as maintain asepsis for the preparation.

12.3-3 Does the C-PEC used for sterile compounding need to be vented to the outside?

Yes. The C-PEC must be externally vented, and the room in which the C-PEC is placed must be externally vented.

12.3-4 Can the C-PEC for sterile compounding be vented into another room instead of to the outside?

No, it must be vented to the outside. You would not want to move potentially hazardous contamination into another interior room.

12.3-5 What should I look for when buying a C-PEC for sterile compounding?

The manufacturer needs to provide documentation that the device meets USP <797> requirements. Be sure to get a BSC that is on the list of NSF Certified Biosafety Cabinetry (http://info.nsf.org/Certified/Biosafety/), which has been independently performance-verified. Standard Class II BSCs that you can purchase will be on this list. If you need a special order BSC for some reason, ask the manufacturer to perform the biological test that they would use for certification of the unit.

12.3-6 I make only two or three sterile chemo preparations a year. Can I use my powder hood in the nonsterile compounding room to do this?

No, that would not provide the aseptic work space required for compounded sterile preparations (CSPs).

12.3-7 Are regular laminar air flow hoods acceptable for compounding with HDs under <800>?

No. Positive pressure laminar air flow hoods intended for preparation of non-hazardous preparations must never be used for preparing HDs. They do not provide the personnel protection required.

12.3-8 I use a positive pressure vertical laminar air flow hood for all CSPs. Will this still be allowed under <800>?

No, nor is it permitted now. Laminar air flow PECs intended for non-hazardous preparation are manufactured in both horizontal and vertical flow. Neither can be used for preparation of antineoplastic HDs. You need to use two different PECs: a positive pressure device for preparation of non-hazardous CSPs and a negative pressure device (e.g., a BSC or CACI) for preparation of hazardous CSPs.

12.3-9 Do I need a separate BSC for non-antineoplastic HDs?

You need to use a BSC or CACI for the preparation of antineoplastic HDs. How you handle your non-antineoplastic HDs depends on your Assessment of Risk. Most organizations will elect to prepare their non-antineoplastic and reproductive hazards in a different device than the antineoplastic agents. You could consider a separate BSC or CACI for it, or you could—if you define alternative containment strategies and/or work practices in your Assessment of Risk—use the devices you use for non-hazardous CSPs.

12.3-10 Can an acrylic glove box be used for preparation of HDs? It isn't negative pressure (there is no pressure differential), and it isn't vented.

No, that device doesn't meet the definition of a C-PEC nor the requirements for personnel safety.

12.3-11 Can I compound chemo and non-HDs in the same C-PEC?

<800> allows this for occasional use, but it is not ideal. If you compound a non-HD in a BSC or CACI, you need to treat any non-HD with HD precautions. This includes placing the non-HD CSP in a bag as you would do for an antineoplastic CSP and labeling it to require the personal protective equipment (PPE) requirements as you would for an

antineoplastic CSP. This needs to be done because the non-HD has been exposed in an area that is potentially contaminated with HD residue. *Think of the patient risks:* would you want an immunocompromised patient receiving intravenous immunoglobulin (IVIG) to receive a dose potentially contaminated with an antineoplastic drug?

12.3-12 My isolator manufacturer says I don't have to place my CACI in a negative pressure room. Is this compliant with <800>?

No. All C-PECs need to be placed in a room with fixed walls that is negative pressure, vented to the outside, and have the appropriate number of ACPH.

12.3-13 Can I compound non-hazardous CSPs in the anteroom?

If you have a cleanroom suite (positive pressure ISO 7 anteroom opening into a negative pressure ISO 7 buffer room with a BSC or CACI), you could place a laminar air flow workbench (LAFW) or compounding aseptic isolator (CAI) in your anteroom. This is not ideal and will not allow you to batch in that area or to use the full beyond-use dates (BUDs) in <797>. The LAFW or CAI and the surrounding space would need to be designed like a segregated compounding area (see USP <797> for full details), so you would be limited to IVs for single patients (no batches) and a BUD of 12 hours.

12.3-14 Can I batch my chemo pre-meds in the anteroom of my negative pressure IV room?

No. Batching CSPs is more complex than mixing an IV for a single patient. You need to mix batches of non-HD CSPs in an appropriately designed positive pressure cleanroom.

12.3-15 Do isolators need to be vented to the outside if they have HEPA filters on the exhaust?

Yes. All C-PECs used for sterile compounding need to be vented to the outside. HD residue can be either particles or vapors. You wouldn't want those to be recirculated into an internal room.

12.3-16 Can I place a regular hood in my negative pressure cleanroom to mix pre-meds?

No. The C-PECs placed in a negative pressure buffer room need to be negative pressure devices (BSCs or CACIs).

12.3-17 USP <800> states that a LAFW cannot be used for compounding antineoplastic HDs. So, can a LAFW or CAI be used for compounding a non-antineoplastic HD?

It depends on your Assessment of Risk. You may exempt compounding of non-antineoplastics and reproductive risks from the requirement to be compounded in a negative pressure PEC if you define and implement alternative containment strategies and/or work practices. Most organizations will compound conventionally manufactured dosage forms of the drugs listed in Tables 2 and 3 of the NIOSH list of HDs in a positive pressure LAFW or CAI, but that must be included in your Assessment of Risk.

12.3-18 Is it true that a CACI must now be installed in a segregated room? This was different from USP <797>, where if the CACI met certain air cleanliness requirements it could stand alone.

That is correct. All PECs used for HD compounding must be placed in a room with fixed walls, under negative pressure room, vented to the outside, with an appropriate number of ACPH. To use the full BUDs allowed in <797>, a minimum of 30 ACPH are needed. For a C-SCA, a minimum of 12 ACPH are needed, but only a 12-hour BUD can be used in that case.

12.3-19 Must CACIs be located in a negative pressure room?

Since the 2008 revision of USP <797>, CACIs have been required to be located in a negative pressure room with 12 ACPH, unless the low volume exemption was applicable. In USP <800>, the CACI must be in a negative pressure room, and it must be vented to the outside of the building.

12.3-20 I have a CACI in a negative room, but it is not a cleanroom. Is this still OK with USP <800> requirements?

The room needs to meet the requirements of a C-SCA: room with fixed walls, negative pressure between 0.01-0.03" wc, vented to the outside, and at least 12 ACPH. The CACI must meet the device requirements listed in USP <797>. The BUDs of preparations made in this area are limited to 12 hours.

12.3-21 I have a CACI in a room that meets the requirements for a C-SCA. Can I still use the full BUDs listed in USP <797>?

No. CSPs mixed in a C-SCA are limited to a 12-hour BUD. It doesn't matter if you use a BSC or a CACI; a 12-hour BUD is the limit.

12.3-22 Are BSCs obsolete? Do I need to get a CACI for my negative pressure cleanroom?

BSCs are not obsolete. Either a BSC or CACI can be used.

12.3-23 What does *class* of a BSC mean?

There are three classes of BSCs:

1. *Class I BSCs*—protect personnel and the environment, but not the preparation. It can be used for nonsterile compounding but not for sterile compounding.
2. *Class II BSCs*—are partial barrier devices that protect personnel, the environment, and the preparation. It is designed for use to compound sterile preparations. It can be used for nonsterile compounding, but a Class I BSC is a more economical choice for a unit that is dedicated to nonsterile use. Class II BSCs are further split into types of Class II BSCs. (See next question.)
3. *Class III BSCs*—are designed for use with highly infectious agents. These are the BSCs you see in photos of personnel who work with anthrax and other extreme hazards. It provides the maximum protection for personnel and the environment. Is it not designed for use with routine sterile compounding.

12.3-24 How are the types of Class II BSCs different?

Class II BSCs are designed to protect personnel and the environment and to maintain asepsis of preparations during sterile compounding. The designations have changed over time, so older BSC manufacturer information may use the older terms.

- *Type A1 units* *were formerly called Type A.* They are not acceptable for sterile compounding use.
- *Type A2 units* *were formerly called Type B3.* They recirculate about 70% HEPA-filtered air back into the room. For most facilities, a Class II Type A2 BSC is the best choice for a simple and reliable integration with the ventilation and pressurization requirements of the negative pressure buffer room for sterile compounding.
- *Type B1 units* *exhaust about 30% of their HEPA-filtered air back into the room.* They have more complex venting and ducting requirements than A2 units.
- *Type B2 units* *do not exhaust any air back into the room.* 100% of their HEPA-filtered air is exhausted to the outside. They have more complex venting and ducting requirements than A2 units.
- *Type C units* are under development and may be available in the future.

12.3-25 I thought USP <797> required total exhaust BSCs.

No. The 2008 version of <797> referred to optimal venting; it is not a requirement. Class II Type A2 units provide a simpler, safer, and more reliable engineering control because they are connected through a canopy rather than hard ducting. The air that is recirculated back into the room is 100% HEPA filtered.

12.3-26 I used to have a BSC that was a Class II, Type A2 unit. The exhaust was directly connected to the outside. Recently, my certifier told me I couldn't have this configuration and had to get either a new hood or change to what they term a *canopy* connection. Why?

Class II, Type A2 BSCs are designed to vent some of the HEPA-filtered air to the outside and allow some of the HEPA-filtered air back into the room. In 2002, NSF/ANSI (which is the organization that oversees BSCs) changed their Standard 49 *Biosafety Cabinetry: Design, Construction, Performance, and Field Certification*[16] to remove the option of direct-connected Type A cabinets, which had been previously allowed. In 2010, NSF changed the language in standard 49 from *should* to *shall*, making it mandatory that all direct-connected Type A cabinets be converted to a canopy connection. In addition, an alarm requirement was added for canopy-connected Type A cabinets. In late 2015, NSF/ANSI notified all personnel accredited to certify BSCs that they would be in violation of the NSF Code of Ethics if they certify a direct-connected Type A cabinet or a canopy-connected Type A cabinet that does not have an alarm.

This is a safety issue: if the air is ducted directly to the outside and something happens to the vent, the air has nowhere to go except back into the BSC, which would blow back at you. A canopy connection allows the HEPA-filtered air to vent without losing containment.

12.3-27 How do I know that my BSC or CACI is working correctly?

You need to have an alarm on the unit, which would alert you any time the ventilation is not adequate.

CLOSED SYSTEM DRUG-TRANSFER DEVICES *13*

(See Sections 5 and 14 in USP <800>.)

<800> requires the use of CSTDs for administration of antineoplastic HDs, when the dosage form allows. The entity may exempt use of CSTDs with non-antineoplastics or reproductive hazards if included in the Assessment of Risk if alternative containment strategies and/or work practices are identified and implemented.

13.1 What is a *CSTD*?

A *CSTD* or closed system drug-transfer device mechanically prohibits the transfer of environmental contaminants into the system and the escape of hazardous drugs (HDs) or vapor concentrations outside the system.

13.2 Does <800> require the use of CSTDs for compounding HDs?

<800> recommends the use of CSTDs for compounding, but it is not a requirement.

13.3 Do CSTDs have to be used when compounding in a CACI?

Use of CSTDs is recommended—not required—when compounding. It does not matter if the compounding is done in a biological safety cabinet (BSC) or compounding aseptic container isolator (CACI); the recommendation is the same.

13.4 Does <800> require the use of CSTDs for administering HDs?

Antineoplastics must be administered with a CSTD when the dosage form allows. The entity may exempt non-antineoplastics and reproductive hazards if included in the Assessment of Risk.

13.5 Do we need to use CSTDs for drugs such as chloramphenicol?

You need to define it in your Assessment of Risk. You can exempt those agents that are not antineoplastics if you include it in your Assessment of Risk, but you must define and implement alternative containment strategies and/or work practices.

13.6 Is <800> requiring or recommending the use of CSTDs for more than just antineoplastic drugs?

The requirement is for use when administering antineoplastics. You can decide in your Assessment of Risk whether you want to exempt dosage forms of non-antineoplastics or reproductive hazards from the administration requirement, but you must define and implement alternative containment strategies and/or work practices.

13.7 Can I use a CSTD instead of a hood for occasional HD compounding?

No; a CSTD cannot be used as a substitute for the appropriate compounding facilities. It is a supplemental engineering control, not a primary engineering control (PEC).

13.8 USP <797> allows compounding an occasional HD in a BSC in a positive pressure room as long as a CSTD is used. Will this be acceptable under USP <800>?

No. The *low use exemption* allowed in the 2008 USP <797> will be eliminated when USP <800> becomes enforceable on July 1, 2018.

13.9 Are CSTDs approved by the FDA?

Drugs are approved by the U.S. Food and Drug Administration (FDA); the term used for devices is *cleared*. The process is not the same as gaining approval for a drug.

13.10 Does the OMB code that some CSTD suppliers use mean that they are approved by the FDA?

No, granting an OMB code is different from the FDA clearance of the device.

13.11 How do I know if the CSTD we want to use actually works?

National Institute for Occupational Safety and Health (NIOSH) published a draft performance protocol for CSTDs; the public comment period ended in March 2016. Although this is not yet finalized, you could ask the CSTD supplier to provide independent testing results for their device.

13.12 Can nursing use a different CSTD for administration than we do in the pharmacy for compounding?

That may be possible (depending on the CSTD components used), but it is probably not efficient. Nursing and pharmacy should work together to select the most appropriate product and components, to promote safety and efficiency, and to minimize the potential for removal of the device prior to use.

13.13 <800> says "CSTDs known to be physically or chemically incompatible with a specific HD must not be used for that HD."[8] I assume a CSTD could be physically incompatible because of physical dimensions, shape, composition, etc., but how could it be chemically incompatible?

In some situations, the components of a drug interact with the composition of the material used in certain CSTDs.

DESIGN OF COMPOUNDING FACILITIES 14

(See Section 5 in USP <800>.)

APIs of any type of HD and antineoplastic must be compounded using the containment strategies and work practices defined in <800>. An entity's Assessment of Risk may exempt specific dosage forms of those agents listed in the NIOSH hazardous list tables for non-antineoplastics and reproductive hazards if alternative containment strategies and/or work practices are identified and implemented.

14.1 GENERAL INFORMATION

14.1-1 What are the minimum facility requirements for compounding HDs?

Hazardous drugs (HDs) must be compounded in a room that is separate from compounding of non-HDs. The room must have fixed walls, be negative pressure, be vented to the outside, and have the appropriate number of air changes per hour (ACPH). Sterile compounding anterooms and buffer rooms require at least 30 ACPH. Nonsterile compounding areas and containment segregated compounding areas (C-SCAs) require at least 12 ACPH. See **Table 14-1** for minimum facility requirements.

14.1-2 What is an *ACPH*?

ACPH is air changes per hour. Thirty (30) ACPH means that the air in the room is turned over every 2 minutes; 12 ACPH means that the air in the room is turned over every 5 minutes. The air changes are a key element in control of a negative pressure area because it removes hazardous particles and vapors.

14.1-3 What are the significant differences between USP <797> and USP <800> regarding requirements for negative pressure rooms and hoods?

Once USP <797> is revised, there will be no differences because <797> will refer to <800> for issues of HDs. ***Until <797> is revised, some differences are noted below:***

- *Negative pressure requirements*—<797> states that the negative rooms must be at least 0.01" wc negative. <800> defines a range between 0.01 to 0.03" wc.
- *Placement of primary engineering controls (PECs)*—<797> allows placement of a compounding aseptic containment isolator (CACI) outside of a negative room. <800> requires all containment PECs (biological safety cabinets [BSCs] or CACIs) to be in a negative pressure room.

14.1-4 Is there a way to look at the current (allowed by <797>) options versus the upcoming (allowed by <800>) options for placement of chemo hoods in different types of allowable rooms?

See **Table 14-2** for examples of requirements. Note that this is only an *example*; your room does not need to look exactly like it.

TABLE 14-1 Minimum Facility Requirements

See USP <795>, <797>, and <800> for details

	Storage	Sterile Compounding		Nonsterile Compounding
	May be either separate room or HDs may be stored in negative pressure buffer room, C-SCA, or nonsterile compounding room	Cleanroom Suite	C-SCA	Compounding Room
PEC	N/A	BSC or CACI		CVE
Room	Room that is separate from non-hazardous activities, with fixed walls, negative pressure between 0.01-0.03" wc to adjacent area, and externally vented			
Configuration	Single room	Positive pressure anteroom and negative pressure buffer room	Single room	Single room
HEPA-filtered ceiling air	Not required	Required	Not required	Not required
ISO classification	Not required	ISO 7	Not required	Not required
Air changes per hour	12 ACPH	30 ACPH	12 ACPH	12 ACPH

ACPH: air changes per hour; BSC: biological safety cabinet; CACI: compounding aseptic containment isolator; C-SCA: containment segregated compounding area; CVE: containment ventilated enclosure; HDs: hazardous drugs; HEPA: high-efficiency particulate air; ISO: International Standards Organization; PEC: primary engineering control; wc: water column

TABLE 14-2 What Is Currently Allowed by <797> and What Will Be Allowed by <800>

Type of PEC	Placement in Room	Allowed by <797>?	Allowed by <800>?
BSC	Cleanroom suite	Yes	Yes
BSC	C-SCA	C-SCA is not defined in <797>	Yes
BSC	Outside of cleanroom suite or C-SCA	No	No
CACI	Cleanroom suite	Yes	Yes
CACI	C-SCA	C-SCA is not defined in <797>	Yes
CACI	Negative pressure room with minimum of 12 ACPH	Yes	No (needs additional room requirements to meet the design of a C-SCA)

ACPH: air changes per hour; BSC: biological safety cabinet; CACI: compounding aseptic containment isolator; C-SCA: containment segregated compounding area; PEC: primary engineering control

14.1-5 What does *fixed walls* mean?

Fixed walls refers to hard walls of appropriate materials and/or finishing. It cannot be a plastic curtain or strips.

14.1-6 Do the walls have to go from floor to ceiling?

Yes.

14.1-7 Can I use plastic curtains or drapes to define the hazardous room?

No. The room must have fixed walls.

14.1-8 Can I have a room with hard walls and use a plastic drape or strips for the doorway?

No. The room must have a door.

14.1-9 Can modular cleanrooms be used?

Yes, as long as they meet <800> requirements. They must have fixed walls, not plastic curtains.

14.1-10 Must *fixed walls* be totally solid? Is a soft-wall system using a solid steel frame affixed to the floor and ceiling OK?

A flexible wall surface might be OK as long as it is fixed in place, contains the room, and meets the other requirements in <800> such as the ability to withstand the disinfection and cleaning agents required.

14.1-11 How much volume is needed to invest in a negative pressure room? We compound a very low volume of HDs, maybe one or two per week.

There is no *low use* exemption in USP <800>, and it will be removed from USP <797> so the two chapters are in synch. If you do any antineoplastic compounding, you need the proper facilities. The two options in <800> are either a negative pressure cleanroom (positive pressure anteroom opening into a negative pressure buffer room) or a C-SCA, which needs to be negative and meet other requirements listed in <800> but does not need to be an International Standards Organization (ISO) 7 cleanroom.

14.1-12 I have an ISO 7 positive pressure anteroom that opens up into two separate buffer rooms: one ISO 7 positive pressure room for non-hazardous sterile compounding and one ISO 7 negative pressure room for chemo compounding. The hoods and the rooms meet <797> requirements and are certified every 6 months. Do I have to build a new negative pressure cleanroom to meet <800>?

If your negative pressure cleanroom meets <797> requirements and is externally vented, it will meet <800> requirements. Be sure that the negative pressure is in the range of 0.01 to 0.03" wc, which is required by <800>.

14.1-13 How do the PECs and the SECs differ from 797?

They don't. They are the same requirements, as long as storage and compounding occur in negative pressure rooms.

14.1-14 Do we need a separate room to do antineoplastic compounding?

Compounding of antineoplastics and of active pharmaceutical ingredient (API) of any type of HDs needs to be done in a negative room that meets <800> requirements. If you already have a compliant room in which you compound antineoplastics, you do not necessarily need another room. Your Assessment of Risk may exempt certain dosage forms of non-antineoplastics or reproductive hazards from compounding in a negative pressure room. This applies to both nonsterile and sterile compounding.

14.1-15 Do I have to mix my chemo in a C-SCA?

You can mix HDs in either a cleanroom suite (ISO 7 positive pressure anteroom opening into an ISO 7 negative pressure buffer room) or in a C-SCA.

14.1-16 Do nonsterile, non-antineoplastic, hazardous medications need to be compounded/prepared in a negative pressure environment?

It depends on your Assessment of Risk. <800> allows you to perform an Assessment of Risk for specific dosage forms of those drugs that are non-antineoplastic or reproductive hazards. You can exempt the dosage forms from some or all of the containment strategies and/or work practices listed in <800> if you identify and implement alternative containment strategies and/or work practices.

14.1-17 We are in the process of building a pharmacy compounding room for nonsterile compounding only (no sterile compounding). Is it possible to compound both non-hazardous and hazardous mixtures in one compounding room?

No, unless you want to treat all your compounds as hazardous. That is not practical from either a personnel or work flow perspective or appropriate for patients. Why would you want to expose personnel and all your finished preparations to potential HD contamination?

14.1-18 What does *negative pressure* mean?

Negative pressure means the room must be negative to adjacent areas, with a negative pressure between 0.01 and 0.03" wc. The net displacement of air is into the room; more air is removed from the room than delivered to it. Air that is removed from the room must be externally vented and not returned to the heating/ventilating/air conditioning (HVAC) system.

14.1-19 What does *separate* mean?

HD storage and preparation must be separate from non-hazardous storage and preparation. You can combine storage and preparation of HDs, because that is separate from non-hazardous storage and preparation.

14.1-20 Can the negative pressure be greater than 0.03" wc?

For rooms used for sterile compounding, the acceptable range is between 0.01 to 0.03" wc.

14.1-21 Is there a requirement for pressure gauges?

Yes. You must be able to measure the pressure of areas that have a pressure requirement at least daily (preferably continuously) to be able to document the pressure is within the required range.

14.1-22 What does *vented to the outside* mean?

Vented to the outside means vented to the outside of the building. Most municipal codes require venting above the roof of the building.

14.1-23 What does *external venting* mean?

External venting means vented to the outside of the building. Most municipal codes require venting above the roof of the building.

14.1-24 Does the external vent need to go to the roof?

Most municipal codes require venting above the roof of the building in a manner so that it will not be taken back into the air handling system. Ideally, this would be at least 30 feet away from the building intake and at least 10 feet above the roof.

14.1-25 Why is venting to the outside of the building needed?

Venting to the outside eliminates any hazardous particles or vapors from the HDs. The negative space required by <800> minimizes the chance of hazardous contamination. Contamination captured in the negative space needs to be evacuated from that area so the area remains safe for personnel.

14.1-26 What does a *classified room* mean?

Classified rooms are those that meet the required ISO criteria for cleanrooms. Relevant categories are ISO 5 (for C-PECs used for sterile compounding) and ISO 7 (for the anteroom and buffer room for sterile compounding).

14.1-27 What is *unclassified* space?

Unclassified space is an area that does not meet ISO standards for a cleanroom.

14.1-28 What ISO classification is required for a cleanroom?

<800> requires an anteroom and buffer room to meet ISO 7 standards.

14.1-29 What ISO classification is required for a C-SCA?

A C-SCA does not need to be ISO classified.

14.1-30 Can HDs be mixed outside a cleanroom?

Yes, they can be mixed in a C-SCA, but the beyond-use date (BUD) allowed for the preparation is limited to 12 hours. HDs cannot be mixed in areas other than a HD cleanroom or a C-SCA.

14.1-31 I have a non-ISO 7 room with a CACI, 12 ACPH, and negative pressure. Will this environment be acceptable to compound HDs under <800>?

These are the basic elements for a C-SCA. If the C-SCA requirements are met, this will be acceptable in <800>. You will need to limit the BUD of any compounds mixed to 12 hours.

14.1-32 Is a negative pressure room required under <800>?

Except for the dosage forms of non-antineoplastics or reproductive hazards that the entity exempts under an Assessment of Risk, storage and compounding of HDs must occur in a negative pressure room. In all cases, API of any type of HD and any antineoplastic that must be manipulated must be stored and compounded in a negative pressure room.

14.1-33 If I handle only HD liquids or semisolids where no particles, aerosols, or gases are produced, do I still need to compound those HDs in a negative room?

APIs of any type of HD and any antineoplastics need to be compounded in a room that meets the requirements of <800>: fixed walls, negative pressure, vented to the outside, and at least 12 ACPH. Final dosage forms of non-antineoplastics or reproductive hazards may be considered for inclusion in your Assessment of Risk if alternative containment strategies and/or work practices are identified and implemented.

14.1-34 What constitutes a *low volume exemption* from <800> requirements?

<800> does not allow for a low volume exemption. All storage and compounding of HDs—except those specific dosage forms of non-antineoplastics and reproductive hazards exempted by the entity in the Assessment of Risk—need to be compounded in an <800>-compliant negative room.

14.1-35 Why did the allowance for *low volume* chemo sites that was allowed in <797> get removed from <800>?

<800> is designed to protect practitioners and the environment as well as patients. <797> allowed placement of a C-PEC in space that was not negative pressure; that design is not allowed in <800>. All storage and compounding of HDs—except those dosage forms of non-antineoplastics or reproductive hazards that have been exempted by the entity's Assessment of Risk—must be in negative pressure. The negative pressure is a key factor in the containment of HDs.

14.1-36 Is it acceptable to prepare HDs in a BSC or CACI in a positive pressure cleanroom?

No API of any type of HD and no antineoplastic agent that requires manipulation may be prepared in a positive pressure room. A negative pressure room is required.

14.1-37 Do negative pressure rooms protect the employees in the room?

Yes. The negative pressure contains the contamination. This needs to be coupled with appropriate venting of the room to remove any contamination.

14.1-38 Are ACPH calculated using supply air or exhaust air?

Conventional wisdom uses the predominant air to calculate ACPH, but calculations for cleanroom and C-SCAs need to be considered differently.

Predominant air would mean that you would use *supply air* (the air coming into your room) for a positive pressure area and *exhaust air* (the air being removed from your room) for a negative pressure area. However, since USP <797> and <800> are designed to provide an aseptic atmosphere for mixing sterile preparations, a cleanroom anteroom and buffer room both require high-efficiency particulate air (HEPA)-filtered air. For this reason, the supply air needs to be used for the calculation. Because a C-SCA doesn't need to have HEPA-filtered air (it does not need to be ISO classified), the calculation follows the conventional wisdom: *use the exhaust air for the calculation.*

To summarize, calculate the ACPH of compounding facility rooms using this logic:
- *Positive pressure ISO-classified anteroom*—use supply air
- *Negative and positive pressure ISO-classified buffer room*—use supply air
- *Negative pressure (non–ISO-classified) C-SCA*—use exhaust air

14.1-39 If the HDs I use are not volatile, why do I need negative pressure and external venting?

Little information is available on the volatility of these drugs. Some studies have shown that common antineoplastic agents volatilize at room temperature. Additionally, the drugs you use could produce hazardous residue from particles. Negative pressure, external venting, and other facility controls noted in <800> protect personnel.

14.1-40 Does *unclassified room* mean it doesn't meet <800> requirements?

Unclassified means it isn't a cleanroom. A C-SCA can be an unclassified room and still meet <800> requirements.

14.1-41 Do I need an area for compounding nonsterile HDs?

Yes, if you do nonsterile compounding of API of any type of HDs or any antineoplastics. If you do this only occasionally, you can use your sterile compounding C-PEC and containment secondary engineering control (C-SEC) with certain restrictions: no sterile compounding can be done while you are using the room for nonsterile compounding, and the C-PEC must be decontaminated, cleaned, and disinfected prior to using the room for sterile compounding.

14.1-42 *Occasional* nonsterile compounding is a subjective term. How many compounds are *occasional*?

There is no number defined in <800>. Consider this as part of your Assessment of Risk. If you do this every day or even every week, it's probably not occasional. If it's your business plan to provide HD nonsterile compounds, it's not occasional. You need the proper equipment for the compounds you mix.

14.1-43 Where does a sink need to be placed?

In a cleanroom suite, you need to place the sink on the clean side of the anteroom. In a C-SCA, you need to place the sink outside the perimeter around your C-PEC. In either case, the sink needs to be at least 1 meter away from the C-PEC.

14.1-44 Can the sink be outside of the C-SCA?

Think of your work practices. You need to don personal protective equipment (PPE) to cover head, hair, and feet, and then wash your hands. If you can do this immediately outside the C-SCA, the placement of the sink could be immediately outside the C-SCA. Then, you would gown and glove inside the C-SCA.

14.1-45 Why does a sink need to be at least 1 meter away from the hood?

It has to be at least 1 meter away from the hood to minimize the chance of microbial contamination.

14.1-46 Can I turn off my hood when I am not using it?

A C-PEC used for sterile compounding or one used to contribute the negative airflow into the room cannot be turned off. A C-PEC (e.g., a powder hood) used only for nonsterile compounding can be turned off when not being used if it does not contribute to the negative air flow requirements of the room.

14.1-47 Why is there a range for negative pressure?

The negative pressure range needs to be between 0.01 and 0.03" wc. The *low range* is required to make the area negative. The *high range* is required as a limit for how negative the room may be. A room that is too negative can promote contamination entering from adjacent areas. Rooms that are too negative often have issues with ceiling tiles loosening or doors not closing correctly, which contribute to the risk of contamination.

14.1-48 Can the HD (negative) room be accessed through the positive pressure buffer room?

Yes, but this is not an ideal configuration. In this case, unless you have a pass-through chamber that bypasses the positive pressure room, you have to transport HDs through the positive pressure area and transport finished hazardous preparations through the positive pressure area. For such an occurrence, you will need to establish policies and practices that contain the drugs, supplies, and finished preparations while they are being transported through the positive pressure area.

14.1-49 Can I have a pass-through between the positive pressure anteroom and the negative pressure buffer room?

Yes, as long as the pass-through chamber meets the requirement listed in <800> and is included in your semiannual room certification. The certifier needs to confirm the particles that could be swept into the negative pressure buffer room are not compromising air quality.

14.1-50 Can I have a pass-through between the general pharmacy area and the negative pressure buffer room?

Yes, as long as the pass-through chamber meets the requirements listed in <800> and it is included in your semiannual room certification. The certifier needs to confirm the particles that could be swept into the negative pressure buffer room from the pass-through are not compromising air quality.

14.1-51 What are the requirements and recommendations for a pass-through chamber?

A pass-through chamber into negative space needs to be limited in size. A 2' x 2' size is generally used. Anything larger could compromise the integrity of the room. The pass-through chamber must have interlocking doors, so only one side could be opened at a time. It should be stainless steel (so will withstand disinfection and cleaning) and made of tempered glass or other material that will withstand decontamination and cleaning.

14.1-52 Can I have a pass-through refrigerator into the negative pressure buffer room?

No. A pass-through refrigerator cannot be used to open into a negative pressure room. That large a space compromises the air quality and also would be a conduit for microbial contamination.

14.1-53 Can I have a cart pass-through (a roll-up door) open into the negative pressure buffer room?

No. A pass-through of this size would be too large a space and would compromise the air quality.

14.1-54 What kind of finishes do I need to use for floors, walls, and ceilings?

Surfaces of ceilings, walls, floors, fixtures, shelving, counters, and cabinets must be smooth, impervious, free from cracks and crevices, non-shedding, and cleanable. This applies to C-SECs for both nonsterile and sterile compounding areas.

14.2 CERTIFICATION OF PRIMARY AND SECONDARY ENGINEERING CONTROLS

14.2-1 How often does certification of the hoods and rooms need to occur?

Engineering controls used for sterile compounding must be certified every 6 months; this is required for all sterile compounding areas. There is no current requirement in USP <795> to certify engineering controls, but these should be certified every 6 months.

14.2-2 What documents should my certifier reference on certification reports?

The certification of BSCs must include compliance with NSF *NSF–ANSI 49*: Class II (laminar flow) Biosafety Cabinetry.[16] Certification of all C-PECs and C-SECs used for sterile compounding should include compliance with the appropriate Controlled Environment Testing Association (CETA) Application Guides, including the current revision of CAG-003-2006[17] for sterile compounding facilities.

14.3 ANTEROOMS

14.3-1 What is the requirement for an anteroom?

The anteroom portion of a negative pressure cleanroom suite needs to be a room with fixed walls, positive pressure of at least 0.02" wc to the room from which it is entered, meet ISO 7 classification, and have at least 30 ACPH.

14.3-2 Can I make both the anteroom and buffer room negative pressure?

No. The anteroom needs to be positive pressure to prevent microbial contamination from coming into your intravenous (IV) area.

14.3-3 Why does the anteroom to a chemo room need to be ISO 7 and not ISO 8?

The negative pressure buffer room needs to be ISO 7. Because that is negative pressure, the air from the anteroom will enter it when the door is open. For this reason, the anteroom needs to be at least as clean as the buffer room to prevent microbial and other contamination from entering the negative pressure buffer room.

14.3-4 Do negative rooms used only for compounding nonsterile HDs (no sterile compounding) require an anteroom?

No.

14.3-5 Does a C-SCA require an anteroom?

No.

14.4 PRE-STERILIZATION AREAS FOR WEIGHING POWDERS

14.4-1 Where should HD powders be weighed for preparation of sterile HD CSPs?

All HD handling needs to be done in a negative pressure area. If the only negative pressure area you have is the negative pressure buffer room, it needs to be done there. Ideally, it will be done in a C-PEC dedicated for that purpose such as a powder hood. In this case, you need to weigh and handle powders only when no sterile compounding is occurring. The room must be able to comply with ISO 7 while the powder-weighing is occurring.

Ideally, you should have a separate negative pressure room that contains a containment ventilated enclosure (CVE) (e.g., a powder hood). The weighing could occur there, then transport the weighed powder in a closed container into the negative pressure buffer room for compounding. If this weighing room is prior to the anteroom, it must be at least ISO 8. If the weighing room is between the anteroom and the buffer room, it must be at least ISO 7.

14.4-2 Can I weigh powders in a negative pressure anteroom?

The anteroom portion of a cleanroom suite needs to be positive pressure. The positive pressure serves to prevent microbial contamination from entering the buffer room. You cannot make your anteroom negative; it must be positive pressure.

However, if you have a room between the positive anteroom and the negative buffer room and you use this interim space for weighing HD powders, you need to make the interim room negative. It also must be ISO 7 because the air in it needs to be at least as clean as the ISO 7 positive anteroom.

14.5 CONTAINMENT SECONDARY ENGINEERING CONTROLS

14.5-1 What are C-SECs?

The *C-SEC* or containment secondary engineering control is the room in which the C-PEC is placed.

14.5-2 How is a C-SEC in <800> different from a SEC for HDs as described in <797>?

If you are talking about the cleanroom suite, it is the same. <797> describes the required space as an ISO 7 positive pressure anteroom opening into an ISO 7 negative pressure buffer room. That configuration is compliant with both <797> and <800>.

However, there are some other differences between what was and wasn't allowed in <797> and the allowances in <800>:

- <797> allowed only a segregated compounding area for non-hazardous drugs; <800> allows a C-SCA for HD compounding.
- <797> allowed use of a CACI outside of a cleanroom if the manufacturer provided appropriate documentation, as long as it was placed in a negative pressure room with at least 12 ACPH. External venting of the CACI was noted as optimal but not required, and full BUDs as listed in <797> were allowed. The C-SCA allowed in <800> must be externally vented, and only a 12-hour BUD is allowed no matter which PEC—either a BSC or a CACI— is used.

14.5-3 What are the minimum requirements for a room/suite to compound HDs with the full BUDs allowed by <797>?

To use the full BUDs listed in <797>, you need to have an ISO 7 positive pressure anteroom that opens into an ISO 7 negative pressure buffer room. The room must have fixed walls and a door between the anteroom and buffer room. The room must be vented to the outside of the building and have at least 30 ACPH in both the anteroom and the buffer room. HEPA-filtered air is required. <800> describes the air handling and other attributes required. The Controlled Environment Testing Association (CETA) Certification Application Guides (CAGs) describe in detail how those attributes of the room are certified. Your certifier should use them and document that for you in your certification report.

14.5-4 Does the exhaust air from a SEC room need to be HEPA filtered?

No. The PEC exhaust air is HEPA filtered, so the room air does not need to be.

14.5-5 Can a negative pressure room be vented to the outside only through the BSC exhaust?

If the BSC is a Class II Type A2 cabinet, the canopy-connected exhaust provides isolation to the BSC from the general HVAC system. If the BSC is a Class II Type B2 cabinet, an additional room exhaust grill is required to protect the BSC from the HVAC variances.

14.5-6 Can I use plastic curtains to separate the anteroom from the buffer room?

No. Those rooms must have fixed walls.

14.5-7 Does *fixed walls* mean I can't use a modular design?

You can use a modular design as long as it has fixed (solid) walls.

14.5-8 Is a C-SCA different from a C-SEC?

A C-SCA is a type of C-SEC. Either of them is your secondary control—the area where your BSC or CACI is placed. The difference is that the C-SCA does not need to be an ISO 7 cleanroom. Because the C-SCA doesn't have HEPA-filtered air or strict control of particles, full BUDs cannot be assigned; you are limited to a 12-hour BUD.

14.5-9 What are the minimum requirements for a C-SCA, and what are the BUD limits?

A C-SCA must have fixed walls, be 0.01 to 0.03" wc negative to adjacent areas, be vented to the outside of the building, and have at least 12 ACPH. <800> describes the air handling and other attributes required. The CETA CAGs describe in detail how those attributes of the room are certified. Your certifier should use them and document that for you in your certification report.

14.5-10 Why would I choose to build a HD cleanroom instead of a C-SCA?

A cleanroom allows you to mix hazardous preparations and assign the full BUD listed in <797>. HD preparations made in a C-SCA have a maximum BUD of 12 hours. To mix any compounded sterile preparation (CSP) component that starts with a nonsterile component, you must have a cleanroom suite because those preparations cannot be compounded in a C-SCA.

14.5-11 A segregated compounding area in <797> can be used only for low-risk preparations. Is that restriction also in <800>?

No. You can compound low- or medium-risk hazardous preparations in a C-SCA. You cannot compound high-risk preparations in a C-SCA.

14.5-12 Can a negative room be too negative?

Yes. A negative room must be between 0.01 to 0.03" wc negative to adjacent space. If it is more negative than that, you have a much greater potential of having contaminants from adjacent room get into the negative pressure buffer room or C-SCA. You may also find that seals around doors and equipment lose integrity.

14.5-13 The door to my negative buffer room won't stay closed. Why does this happen?

Check the pressure difference between the negative room and adjacent space. You may find that the negative pressure is higher than it should be. The proper range is 0.01 to 0.03" wc negative. Once you exceed that range, often doors won't close, refrigerator doors are hard to open, and ceiling tiles come uncaulked. The reason is because the negative pressure is too great for those doors and seals to work properly.

14.5-14 I have a CACI in a room. Does the room itself need to be negative pressure, or is it enough if the CACI vents to the outside?

The room needs to be negative. All compounding needs to be done in a negative room. The protection of the negative space isn't only for the compounding but also for storage, transporting antineoplastic vials into the CACI, and moving completed HD preparations out of the CACI.

14.5-15 Do ceilings really need to be caulked in place under <800>?

Yes. All the requirements listed for facilities need to be compliant.

14.5-16 Why do I need to place my CACI in a negative room if the manufacturer says I don't have to place it in ISO 7?

There are two different issues here: (1) compounding in negative space and (2) placement of the CACI outside of a cleanroom. All HD compounding needs to be done in a negative room; the type of device—BSC or CACI—doesn't matter. The negative room protects you from contamination when you are compounding. Location of the CACI outside of ISO 7 is an issue both of <797> and <800>. If you find a 12-hour BUD acceptable, you could place the CACI in a C-SCA (which doesn't require ISO-classified air).

14.5-17 Do all HDs have to be compounded in a negative pressure room or just antineoplastic drugs?

It depends on your Assessment of Risk. You must compound the antineoplastic agents in a BSC or CACI in a negative pressure room. If you don't perform an Assessment of Risk, or if your Assessment of Risk determines that you will compound some or all of the non-antineoplastic and/or reproductive hazards as you would antineoplastic agents, then you would have to compound them in a negative pressure room. However, you then need to treat all of those drugs as you would chemo agents, since they could be contaminated with HD residue. More likely, you will want to perform an Assessment of Risk for the non-antineoplastics and reproductive hazards and compound them with the alternative containment strategies you identify.

14.5-18 Is there a statement in <800> about not compounding non-antineoplastic HDs in a negative pressure room?

It's not worded that way. Antineoplastics must be compounded in a negative pressure room. You can perform an Assessment of Risk for agents that are non-antineoplastic and/or reproductive hazards and determine alternative containment strategies and/or work practices for those agents. You may determine that some or all of the non-antineoplastic agents or reproductive hazards can be compounded in a positive pressure room, but you would have to identify what your alternative containment strategies are for dosage forms of those agents.

14.5-19 Are there examples of designs for a C-SEC that I can use to explain the requirements?

See **Figure 14-1** for an example of room requirements. Note that this is only an *example*; your room does not need to look exactly like it.

14.5-20 Should the un-gowning area be inside the negative pressure room or outside of it?

The doffing area should be immediately next to the door where you exit the negative pressure room. You need to doff the gown and outer pair of shoe covers as you are leaving the negative pressure area, so you don't contaminate the positive pressure anteroom with any potential HD contaminants.

14.5-21 Can a CVE used for non-hazardous compounding and a separate CVE used for hazardous compounding be in the same C-SCA?

That is not a practical approach because you would then need to treat all of your non-hazardous preparations as hazardous.

14.6 CONTAINMENT SEGREGATED COMPOUNDING AREAS

14.6-1 What is a C-SCA?

A *C-SCA* or containment segregated compounding area is a type of secondary engineering control but does not require HEPA air or ISO classification. It does have to be a room with fixed walls, be between 0.01 to 0.03" wc negative to adjacent areas, be vented to the outside, and have at least 12 ACPH. You should define a perimeter around the BSC or CACI. (This serves a similar purpose as an anteroom in a cleanroom suite.) A sink needs to be either inside the room (but outside the perimeter around BSC or CACI) or immediately available outside the room.

14.6-2 Can the C-SCA be an *area* and not a *room*?

No. It must be a room with fixed walls.

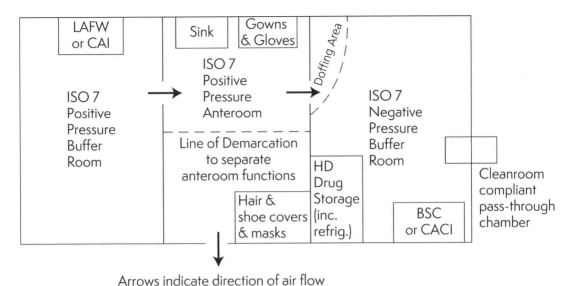

FIGURE 14-1 Example of Cleanroom Suite, Including a Containment Secondary Engineering Control

14.6-3 What is the difference between a negative pressure cleanroom and a C-SCA?

The negative pressure cleanroom has HEPA-filtered air, meets at least ISO 7 classification, and has a separate anteroom and buffer room. The C-SCA does not require those characteristics.

14.6-4 Is a C-SCA in <797> the same as a C-SCA in <800>?

Not from a design perspective, but it serves a similar purpose: to allow CSPs to be compounded in an area that isn't a cleanroom as long as only a short BUD is assigned. The design of a C-SCA has more and different requirements than a SCA used for non-hazardous preparations. The C-SCA must be a room with fixed walls, be under negative pressure, be vented to the outside, and have at least 12 ACPH.

14.6-5 Does a C-SCA have to be negative pressure?

Yes. All compounding of antineoplastics must be done in a negative pressure room.

14.6-6 Does a C-SCA have to contain HEPA-filtered ceiling air?

No. HEPA-filtered air is not required in a C-SCA.

14.6-7 Does a C-SCA require an anteroom?

No, but a perimeter should be defined around the BSC or CACI. No water sources or drains should be inside the perimeter.

14.6-8 How big does the perimeter in a C-SCA need to be?

You can define it. You need enough space for the BSC or CACI, a chair (if you use a chair) for the person compounding, and some additional space so that the entire compounding procedure and person compounding fit inside the perimeter.

14.6-9 What is the purpose of the perimeter in a C-SCA? What can be inside of the perimeter? What needs to be outside the perimeter?

The perimeter around the BSC or CACI serves a similar purpose as the division between the anteroom and the buffer room in a cleanroom suite. It defines the area where compounding occurs. *It's probably easier to define what **cannot** be in the perimeter*: no sink or other water sources, no floor drains, no storage shelving, or anything else extraneous to the final compounding activities.

14.6-10 Is there an example of a design for a C-SCA that I can use to explain the requirements?

See **Figure 14-2** for an example of room requirements. Note that this is only an *example*; your room does not need to look exactly like it.

14.6-11 Should the un-gowning area be inside the negative pressure room or outside of it?

The doffing area should be immediately next to the door where you exit the negative pressure room. You need to doff the gown and outer pair of shoe covers as you are leaving the negative pressure area, so you don't contaminate adjacent areas with any potential HD contaminants.

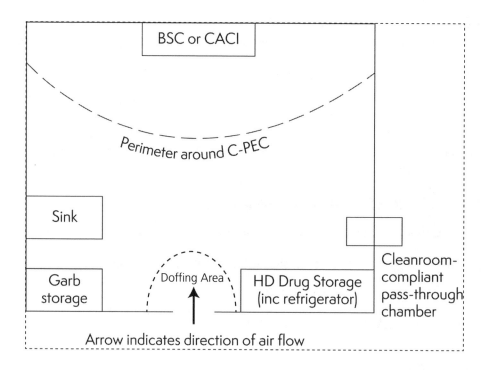

FIGURE 14-2 Example of Containment Segregated Compounding Area

14.7 PASS-THROUGH CHAMBERS

14.7-1 What is a *pass-through chamber*?

A *pass-through chamber* is a box-like structure in a wall between areas in a cleanroom suite or C-SCA. It needs to be limited in size—most are about 2′ high x 2′ wide—and are useful between the main pharmacy and negative pressure buffer room, or between the main pharmacy and the C-SCA. You use this chamber to pass supplies into the negative pressure room and/or completed preparations out of the negative pressure room.

14.7-2 Are there specific structural requirements for a pass-through?

Yes. The chamber must be included in the semi-annual certification to be sure that it isn't compromising the air quality of the negative room. Appropriate cleanroom pass-throughs should be made of stainless steel and tempered glass (or other similar material) and must have interlocking doors (so only one door can be opened at a time).

14.7-3 How can I be sure a pass-through chamber isn't allowing particles into the chemo room?

The pass-through chamber needs to be tested during your semi-annual certification. The certifier needs to be sure that the integrity of the unit is intact.

14.7-4 Does a pass-through chamber into a chemo room need to be negative pressure?

Not necessarily. Because of the limited size and need for interlocking doors, the pass-through should not compromise the integrity of the room. It's less disruptive than when you open the door to enter the room, because the opening is smaller.

14.7-5 Is a pass-through chamber the same as a pass-through window?

No. A window that opens or slides is not appropriate. It has to be a pass-through designed for use in a cleanroom, including use of interlocking doors.

14.7-6 Is a pass-through chamber the same as what I have in my compounding isolator?

No. A compounding isolator has an ante-chamber that is the transition between the room and the workspace of the compounding isolator. Both are often called pass-throughs, but they are different.

14.7-7 Is a pass-through chamber the same as a cart pass-through or a pass-through refrigerator?

No. The difference is the size. A pass-through chamber that you would use into a negative compounding area must be limited in size; most are about 2′ wide x 2′ high. That is small enough so it won't compromise the air quality in the negative room. <800> does not permit large pass-throughs such as a cart pass-through or a pass-through refrigerator. They are too large in size and would compromise the air quality in the negative room. Additionally, they are an infection control risk, since any microbial contamination could be swept into the negative room because of the air pressure difference.

14.7-8 Can I place a pass-through chamber between the main pharmacy and the chemo room?

Yes. This works very well as long as it is considered in the air flow and air quality of the negative room. It needs to be a limited size pass-through and include interlocking doors so only one side can be opened at a time.

14.7-9 Can I place a pass-through chamber between the anteroom and the chemo room?

Yes, as long as it is considered in the air flow and air quality of the negative room. It needs to be a limited size pass-through and include interlocking doors so only one side can be opened at a time.

14.7-10 Can I place a cart pass-through into the chemo room?

No. That size would be too large and too much of a risk to compromise the air quality in the room.

14.7-11 Can I place a pass-through refrigerator between the main pharmacy and the chemo room?

No. That size would be too large and too much of a risk to compromise the air quality in the room. It also would present a risk of microbial contamination being swept into the negative room by the air pressure difference.

14.7-12 Can I place a pass-through refrigerator between the anteroom and the chemo room?

No, that size would be too large and too much of a risk to compromise the air quality in the room. It also would present a risk of microbial contamination being swept into the negative room by the air pressure difference between positive and negative space.

14.7-13 Can I place a pass-through refrigerator between a negative HD storage room and my negative buffer room?

No, that size would be too large and too much of a risk to compromise the air quality in the room.

14.8 REFRIGERATOR AND FREEZER PLACEMENT

14.8-1 Can I put a refrigerator or freezer in my negative cleanroom or C-SCA?

Yes. Antineoplastics must be stored in a negative pressure room, including those that must be refrigerated or frozen. If there are dosage forms of non-antineoplastics or reproductive hazards that you have not exempted in your Assessment of Risk, they may also need to be stored in a negative pressure room. You can have a separate negative pressure storage room dedicated only to storage, or you can store your HDs used for sterile compounding in your negative pressure buffer room or negative pressure C-SCA, as long as you have adequate room to do so and as long as the room can meet the certification parameters.

14.8-2 How can we put bulk storage and refrigerators in the buffer zone? I thought <797> was against it.

There is no such restriction in <797>. The test is if the room will certify with whatever equipment and supplies are in it. You don't want to use the buffer room as a bulk storage room for external containers or corrugated cardboard, but limited stock is fine as long as you have adequate space and the room can meet the certification parameters. If you have a refrigerator in your buffer room or C-SCA, an exhaust placed behind the refrigerator's compressor will serve to remove any particles generated.

14.8-3 Are we allowed to have a refrigerator in the negative pressure room to store refrigerated antineoplastics?

Yes.

14.8-4 Do I have to place a refrigerator in the compounding area?

If you have antineoplastics that need to be refrigerated, you must have that refrigerator in the negative area. If you don't have HDs that require refrigeration, you do not need to place a refrigerator there.

14.8-5 Does USP <800> mention anything about a pass-through refrigerator for chemo?

Yes. Pass-through refrigerators are prohibited.

14.9 ELIMINATION OF LOW VOLUME EXEMPTION FROM 2008 USP <797>

14.9-1 I have been using the exemption in <797> for low volume of chemo preparations, so my chemo hood is in my regular buffer room. I don't see this listed in <800>. Has the requirement changed?

The requirement has changed; this is *not* allowed in <800>. All compounding must be done in a negative pressure room.

14.9-2 I compound only one or two chemos a week. I have only one IV room, and it's positive pressure. Why can't I continue to compound them in my IV room?

<800> requires antineoplastics to be compounded in a negative pressure room. This is for your safety as well as that of your patients and the environment. What if you drop a vial on the way to the BSC or CACI? The contents of that vial are now spread all over your IV room

because it's positive pressure. After you open the door, the particles could be pushed out into your main pharmacy due to the pressure difference.

14.9-3 I cannot get approval to build a negative pressure cleanroom. What are my options?

Because <800> will now be an enforceable chapter, this may increase your influence to get approval for a negative pressure cleanroom. If you can work with a short BUD of 12 hours, you could consider use of a C-SCA, which isn't as expensive to build because it doesn't require HEPA-filtered air or ISO classification. In any case, you must have the proper facility if you need to mix antineoplastics for your patients.

14.10 OTHER ATTRIBUTES FOR DESIGNING A HD COMPOUNDING AREA

14.10-1 What type of sink do I need, and where should it be placed?

Be sure your sink is big enough and deep enough so you can wash your hands without splashing adjacent counters. Stainless steel is best; ceramic sinks are prone to chipping, so they become an infection control risk. Your sterile compounding sink must be limited to uses involving sterile compounding. Never bring in any items that could adversely affect your particle control or promote contamination.

14.10-2 Can I put shelving in my cleanroom or C-SCA?

Yes, but the area should not be used for bulk storage. The items on shelving in your anteroom, buffer room, or C-SCA should be limited to what you need for that day or two.

14.10-3 Can I put a refrigerator in my cleanroom or C-SCA?

Yes. Your refrigerated antineoplastic agents need to be stored in a negative room. As long as you have adequate space in your negative pressure buffer room or C-SCA and the room certifies, it is a logical and convenient place to store your antineoplastic drugs. <800> recommends placement of an exhaust grill behind the refrigerator in an ISO Class 7 room.

14.10-4 Can I put a printer in my cleanroom or C-SCA?

Yes. This is not an issue of <800> but one of <797>, which allows placement of a printer or other necessary equipment as long as the equipment does not adversely affect the operation of the room.

14.10-5 What type of finishes for the floors, walls, and ceilings do I need?

All of that is defined in <797>.[18] They need to be "smooth, impervious, free from cracks and crevices, and non-shedding."[8] They need to withstand the disinfecting and cleaning solutions and procedures used.

14.10-6 Shouldn't all surfaces for HD compounding (sterile and nonsterile) be "smooth, impervious, free from cracks and crevices, and non-shedding"? Why is this listed only under Nonsterile Compounding in USP <800>?

It is listed in USP <797> so is already required for sterile compounding facilities. No similar wording is in the current version of USP <795> for nonsterile compounding; therefore, it is listed in USP <800> as a requirement.

14.10-7 Do I need to have the BSC, CACI, or room on emergency power?

The ventilation systems should have an uninterrupted power source (UPS) to maintain the negative pressure. Some accreditation organization standards also require emergency power for PECs (often called *hoods* in those standards).

COMPOUNDING HAZARDOUS DRUGS   15

(See Section 13 in USP <800>.)

APIs of any type of HDs and antineoplastics must be compounded using the containment strategies and work practices defined in <800>. An entity's Assessment of Risk may exempt specific dosage forms of those agents listed in the NIOSH hazardous list tables for non-antineoplastics and reproductive hazards if alternative containment strategies and/or work practices are identified and implemented.

15.1 What type of policies should I have?

USP <800> details specific policies that must be included. See **Exhibit 15-1**. Your state, accreditation organization, or other agency may require additional policies.

15.2 In 2006, ASHP published guidelines on handling HDs, including a detailed process for decontaminating the final prepared CSP. Does <800> require use of the same steps?

The *ASHP Guidelines on Handling Hazardous Drugs*[3] contains many suggested procedural details. USP <800> leaves development of policy details to each entity. The ASHP document is a valuable resource for development of policies.

15.3 What are good sources to review for developing policies?

In addition to the list of required policies included in USP <800> (see Exhibit 15-1), review these sources:
- *ASHP Guidelines on Handling Hazardous Drugs*[3]
- *NIOSH Alert* on *Preventing Occupational Exposure to Antineoplastic and Other Hazardous Drugs in Health Care Settings*[4]
- Critical Point Pearls of Knowledge archives[19]
- Joint Commission Resources Hazardous Drug Toolkit[20]

15.4 What is an *API*?

An API or active pharmaceutical ingredient is defined by USP <800> as "any substance or mixture of substances intended to be used in the compounding of a drug preparation, thereby becoming the active ingredient in that preparation and furnishing pharmacological activity or other direct effect in the diagnosis, cure, mitigation, treatment, or prevention of disease in humans and animals or affecting the structure and function of the body."[8] It's informally referred to as *powder* or *raw material*.

(questions continued on p. 112)

EXHIBIT 15-1

Policies Required and Recommended in USP <800>

- List of HDs and dosage forms handled
  - Review of list every 12 months
  - Add new agents and dosage forms when used
- Assessment of Risk
  - Antineoplastics that require only packaging or counting, non-antineoplastics, and reproductive hazards can be included
  - Include
    - Type of HD
    - Dosage form
    - Risk of exposure
    - Packaging
    - Manipulation
  - Alternative containment and/or work practices used to exempt HDs from full <800> requirements
  - Review and document at least every 12 months
- Designated Person
  - Qualification and training
  - Responsibilities include
    - Develop and implement policies and procedures
    - Oversee entity compliance with USP <800> and other applicable laws, regulations, and standards
    - Ensure competency of personnel
    - Ensure environmental control of the storage and compounding areas
    - Understand rationale for risk-prevention policies and risks to personnel
    - Report potentially hazardous situations to the management team
    - Monitor the facility
    - Maintain reports of testing/sampling performed in the facility and act on the results
- Hazard Communication program
  - Written confirmation acknowledging understanding of risks
- Occupational safety program
  - Medical surveillance
    - Routine
    - Following acute exposure
- Personnel training
  - Compliance with appropriate USP standards for compounding, including <795> and <797>
  - Overview of the entity's list of HDs and their risks
  - Review of the entity's SOPs related to handling of HDs
  - Proper use of PPE
  - Proper use of equipment and devices
  - Response to known or suspected HD exposure
  - Spill management
  - Proper disposal of HDs and bulk and trace contaminated materials

EXHIBIT 15-1 (cont'd)

- Personnel responsibilities
  - Understand the fundamental practices and precautions
  - Continually evaluate procedures and the quality of final HDs to prevent harm to patients
  - Minimize exposure to personnel
  - Minimize contamination of the work and patient care environment
  - Documented competence
- Designation of HD areas
  - Signs
  - Restricted access to authorized personnel only
- Facility and engineering controls
  - Receiving and unpacking
    - In neutral or negative area
    - Not in positive area
  - Storage
    - Room with fixed walls, negative pressure, externally vented, 12 ACPH
    - Prevent spillage or breakage if container falls
    - Not stored on the floor
    - Meet applicable safety precautions
    - Any HD requiring manipulation other than counting or repackaging of final dosage form and any antineoplastic HD must be stored separately from non-HD stock
    - Refrigerator and/or freezer
  - Nonsterile compounding
    - Room with fixed walls, negative pressure, externally vented, at least 12 ACPH
    - Surfaces of ceilings, walls, floors, fixtures, shelving, counters, and cabinets must be smooth, impervious, free from cracks and crevices, non-shedding, and able to withstand decontamination and cleaning
    - C-PEC and room
      - PEC must be operated continuously if it supplies some or all of the negative pressure in the C-SEC
    - Sink and eyewash location—no closer to C-PEC than 1 meter
    - If in same C-SEC as C-PEC for sterile compounding, cannot compound while sterile compounding occurring
  - Sterile compounding
    - Room with fixed walls, negative pressure, externally vented, at least 12 ACPH for C-SCA or at least 30 ACPH for cleanroom suite (positive pressure anteroom plus negative pressure buffer room)
    - Line of demarcation for donning/doffing PPE
    - Surfaces of ceilings, walls, floors, fixtures, shelving, counters, and cabinets must be smooth, impervious, free from cracks and crevices, non-shedding, and able to withstand decontamination and cleaning
    - C-PEC and room
      - Must be operated continuously
    - Sink and eyewash location—no closer to C-PEC than 1 meter
  - Uninterrupted power source for negative pressure ventilation system

EXHIBIT 15-1 (cont'd)

- Certification of C-PEC and C-SEC
    - C-PECs for nonsterile compounding
    - C-PECs for sterile compounding must be certified at least every 6 months
    - C-SECs for sterile compounding must be certified at least every 6 months
    - Pass-through chambers must be included in the certification
- Beyond-use dates
    - Refer to <795> for nonsterile compounds
    - Refer to <797> for sterile compounds
- Closed system drug-transfer devices
    - Use for compounding
    - Use for administering
- Hand hygiene
- Proper use of PPE
    - Gloves
    - Gowns
    - Head and hair covers
    - Shoe covers
    - Sleeve covers
    - Eye and face protection
    - Respiratory protection
        - Fit testing
    - Disposal of used PPE
    - Decontamination of reusable PPE
- Labeling HDs
- Packaging HDs
    - Use of clean equipment and supplies
    - Decontamination of outer surfaces of finished compounds (nonsterile and sterile)
    - Restriction—no use of automated counting or packaging machines
- Transporting HDs
    - Appropriate shipping containers and insulating materials
    - Applicable federal, state, and local information
- Dispensing HDs
- Administering HDs
    - Use of CSTDs
    - Additional PPE when manipulating outside of ventilated cabinet
- Safe work practices
    - Receiving—assessing shipping containers
    - Use of C-PECs
    - Method to transport HDs in and out of negative pressure room
    - Method to transport HD waste out of negative pressure room
    - Priming IV tubing with non-HD solution
    - Crushing in plastic pouch

EXHIBIT 15-1 (cont'd)

- Decontamination and cleaning
  - Deactivation
    - Solutions used and procedure
  - Decontamination
    - Solutions used and procedure
  - Cleaning
    - Solutions used and procedure
  - Disinfecting
    - Solutions used and procedure
- Environmental wipe sampling
- Waste segregation and disposal
  - Applicable federal, state, and local information and organizational policy
- Spill management
  - Responsibility based on size and scope of spill
  - Use of full-facepiece, chemical cartridge-type respirators if the spill kit capacity is exceeded or if there is known or suspected airborne exposure to vapors or gases
  - Location of spill kits
  - Contents of spill kits
  - Spill response team
  - Documentation of spill

ACPH: air changes per hour; C-PEC: containment primary engineering control; C-SCA: containment segregated compounding area; C-SEC: containment secondary engineering control; CSTDs, closed system drug-transfer devices; HDs, hazardous drugs; IV, intravenous; PPE: personal protective equipment; SOPs: standard operating procedures

15.5 Is it OK to compound non-HDs in the negative pressure hood and room?

Any non-hazardous drug (HD) you place in the negative pressure compounding area needs to be treated as a HD because it could be contaminated with HD residue. If you are talking about making chemo pre-meds in your biological safety cabinet (BSC), details in USP <800> describe the labeling you have to use on that agent.

15.6 Do nonsterile, non-antineoplastic hazardous medications need to be compounded and prepared in a negative pressure environment?

It depends on your Assessment of Risk. USP <800> allows you to exempt certain dosage forms of those agents that are not antineoplastic if you identify alternative containment strategies and/or work practices.

15.7 For non-antineoplastic hazardous oral solutions, does drawing up patient-specific doses from a bulk bottle need to be done in a negative pressure room?

This is a manipulation of a HD, so containment strategies are necessary. You have to define them in your Assessment of Risk.

15.8 If I need to crush tablets to make a solution, where do I do that?

If it is an antineoplastic agent, it needs to be done in a containment primary engineering control (C-PEC) in a negative pressure room. If it is a non-antineoplastic or a reproductive hazard, you can define alternative containment strategies and/or work practices in your Assessment of Risk.

15.9 Can I compound nonsterile HDs in an open room?

No, if you mean in a general compounding area also used for non-hazardous compounding. All compounding of HDs needs to be done in a C-PEC (hood) located in a containment secondary engineering control (C-SEC) (room) unless those types of HDs permitted by your Assessment of Risk—limited to non-antineoplastics or reproductive HDs—have alternative containment strategies and/or work practices.

15.10 Do I have to package methotrexate tablets in a CVE?

Not necessarily, if you address this in your Assessment of Risk. However, if you have a containment ventilated enclosure (CVE), consider using it for packaging oral antineoplastics.

15.11 Do I have to split methotrexate tablets in a CVE?

Splitting tablets is manipulation of the dosage form, so it must occur in a C-PEC (hood) located in a C-SEC (room). If you have a C-PEC used for nonsterile compounding (e.g., a powder hood), use it. If you have only a sterile negative pressure room with a BSC or compounding aseptic containment isolator (CACI) because you rarely need a device for nonsterile compounding, you can use the BSC or CACI. No sterile compounding can occur in that room while manipulation of the nonsterile drug (i.e., methotrexate tablets) is occurring. You need to decontaminate, clean, and disinfect the C-PEC prior to resuming sterile compounding activities.

15.12 I mix about 200 grams of a hormone cream at one time but dispense it in 30-gram containers. After I make the 200 grams, can I store it outside the negative pressure area and place 30 grams in a container when I need to?

If you always dispense in 30-gram containers, why not package them when you mix the 200 grams? Then, you will have finished dosage forms ready for dispensing and could develop alternative containment practices as part of your Assessment of Risk. For example, you could place each 30-gram container in a plastic bag, place them all in a designated bin, and store them in your general storage area. The container and the plastic overwrap could be designated as part of your alternative containment strategies.

15.13 We have a compliant BSC in a compliant cleanroom for HDs. Once or twice a year, we need to weigh out HD APIs in our BSC. Is this OK?

Yes, as long as there is no sterile compounding occurring while you are doing it; the room maintains International Standards Organization (ISO) 7 under operating conditions; and you decontaminate, clean, and disinfect the hood after weighing and before sterile compounding resumes.

15.14 Will USP <800> allow an exemption for nursing to draw up methotrexate in the emergency department?

No. This is an antineoplastic and needs to be prepared under conditions that protect the healthcare worker.

15.15 When is a HD not a HD? When I dissolve it in liquid or add it to a cream or ointment, does it become non-hazardous?

No, it is still a HD. A preparation with any hazardous component is a HD.

15.16 When is a compounded topical cream able to leave the negative pressure area?

It can leave the negative pressure area when it is in a finished dosage form, such as the container in which it will be dispensed. Decontaminate the outside of the container prior to removal from the negative pressure area.

15.17 Is it OK to prepare HDs in the same Class II Type B2 BSC where biological preparations occur?

Is the BSC in a positive pressure room and dedicated for use with biologics? That could occur for those biologics, which are not HDs. If that is what you mean, it would not be appropriate to use that BSC for HDs because the BSC is not in a negative room.

Is the BSC in a negative room? If that is the case, are you asking if all biologics need to be prepared under conditions used for HDs? Some biologics are listed in the National Institute for Occupational Safety and Health (NIOSH) list of HDs.[5] Those on the list need to be compounded with all the containment strategies and work practices listed in <800>.

15.18 What is the best way to handle bacillus Calmette-Guérin?

Bacillus Calmette-Guérin or BCG is a HD that is a live bacillus. The package insert contains special precaution information, but it pre-dates USP <800> so the information is not complete from a contemporary standpoint. Ideally, BCG should be compounded in a separate BSC in a separate negative pressure buffer room that is restricted for use with BCG. In most facilities, that is not a practical solution. The next best option is to work with your physician and nursing staff to schedule all BCG patients at the end of the day. Complete other HD preparation prior to working with BCG. Prepare the BCG, then do a complete decontamination and cleaning of the BSC and negative pressure room. Let the room rest overnight, allowing multiple purges of the room air.

15.19 Why do I have to doff garb in the chemo room?

Personal protective equipment (PPE) is used to protect personnel from potential contamination. You wouldn't want to spread that contamination by walking into a positive pressure area. Therefore, you need to remove your gown, outer gloves, and outer pair of shoe covers as you leave the negative pressure room prior to entering the positive pressure area.

15.20 Can the check of chemo items occur in the anteroom, or does it need to occur in the buffer room?

That depends on your work processes. There is no specific requirement to perform the check in a particular spot.

15.21 Why do I have to label non-chemo meds made in a BSC with PPE precautions?

Ideally, a C-PEC should be used to prepare only HDs. However, in some cases—such as a chemo infusion center where only a BSC is available—USP <800> allows occasional preparation of non-HDs in the C-PEC. Because the drugs and supplies exposed in a C-PEC could be contaminated with a HD, any compounded sterile preparation (CSP) made in that device must be assumed to be contaminated. Therefore, PPE precautions must be used to protect personnel and patients.

If this is your practice, evaluate the risks to personnel and patients. This is particularly important if your infusion center cares for a mix of oncology and other patients. Would you want an immunocompromised patient's intravenous (IV) immune globulin contaminated with cyclophosphamide? Consider eliminating this possibility by mixing non-HDs in a separate PEC.

15.22 Why do I need to use a plastic-backed preparation mat for compounding HDs?

USP <800> recommends, but does not require, the use of a mat. ***The mat serves several purposes:*** protects the desk of the C-PEC from contamination, defines a compounding area, and is useful when gathering up used supplies for discarding after compounding.

15.23 Should the plastic-backed preparation mat be replaced each time the hood is cleaned?

Yes. You would not want to place a potentially contaminated mat back onto a decontaminated surface.

15.24 Does the plastic-backed mat need to be sterile when used for sterile compounding?

No. Similar to other supplies brought into the C-PEC (e.g., packaging of needles and syringes), it does not need to be sterile.

15.25 Is it OK to spray alcohol?

No. Avoid spraying anything in a HD area. Spraying could aerosolize HD residue.

15.26 How frequently should we change the spray bottles of cleaners?

Do not use spray bottles in your HD areas. Spraying can aerosolize HD or residue. Additionally, do not refill bottles for cleaners unless the manufacturer information supports that practice. Use the manufacturer's information for the stability time of the solution.

15.27 How should alcohol be applied in the C-PEC if I can't use a spray?

Purchase or prepare pre-saturated alcohol low-lint wipes.

15.28 Is it OK to use pre-saturated gauze to disinfect vials?

Do not use gauze or any material that sheds when compounding sterile preparations. Use purchased or prepared low-lint wipes that are saturated with the solution you use for decontaminating and disinfecting vials.

HD vials need to be decontaminated prior to placement in the storage area. Then they need to be disinfected prior to placement into the C-PEC.

See Section 21, Decontamination and Cleaning, for more details, and see <797> for practices to use for all sterile compounding.

15.29 Are CSTDs required in an isolator?

USP <800> recommends, not requires, use of closed system drug-transfer devices (CSTDs) when compounding. (CSTDs are required when administering antineoplastic HDs when the dosage form allows.) USP <800> does not differentiate between requirements or recommendations for compounding based on the type of C-PEC used.

15.30 Can corrugated cardboard be used in a negative pressure cleanroom?

No. Any outside shipping container or any corrugated cardboard must be prohibited from placement in any anteroom, cleanroom, or C-SCA. Those materials shed particles and could contribute to microbial contamination.

15.31 Is there a disposable mortar and pestle that can be used for compounding HDs?

Several companies make disposable compounding supplies that can be used instead of reusable items.

15.32 Can I use alcohol gel instead of washing my hands when I take off my gloves?

No. Wash your hands with soap and water after removing gloves. The friction of rubbing your hands helps to remove any potential contamination.

15.33 Do I have to record lot numbers for every chemo?

USP <800> does not deal with issues that apply to general compounding issues. For those requirements, see USP <795> for *Compounding Nonsterile Preparations*[21] and USP <797> for *Compounding Sterile Preparations*. Your state, accreditation organization, or health system may have additional requirements.

15.34 Is a different type of technique used for compounding HDs than used for regular compounding?

Yes. A negative pressure technique is used for compounding HDs, which prevents overpressurization of vials that could cause vial leakage and contamination (see **Exhibit 15-2**).

15.35 Does negative pressure technique have to be used if closed CSTDs are used for compounding?

In most cases, no. Check the instructions for the specific CSTD to determine it. This is an advantage of using a CSTD for compounding.

15.36 What is the recommendation for HDs that are needed emergently (e.g., valproic acid, fosphenytoin)? Should they be compounded in the pharmacy's BSC rather than in the Emergency Department or intensive care unit?

There are several issues here: the need for stat meds for urgent patient situations, ability to provide ready-to-use dosage forms (which is more of a regulatory and accreditation issue), and types of HDs. Fosphenytoin is listed in the non-antineoplastic table of the 2016 NIOSH list of HDs[5]; valproic acid is listed in the reproductive hazards. After performing an Assessment of Risk, you might determine alternative containment strategies you could employ.

Things to consider: the ability for pharmacy to mix them, provision of ready-to-use dosage forms (which would be pharmacy-prepared rather than purchased in these cases), and the containment strategies and/or work practices that you could employ if pharmacy is not able to provide them in time for stat doses.

15.37 If <800> requires compounding in negative pressure rooms, why is there a need to discuss compounding outside of the proper facility?

Some antineoplastic agents may need to be prepared outside of proper engineering controls. This should be done only if there is no way to prepare it for administration with all the containment requirements listed in <800>, and if it is needed for patient use during procedures. Items like mitomycin for ophthalmic use, BCG for bladder irrigations, or methotrexate for ectopic pregnancy present challenging situations. If this can be compounded (or prepared for administration) in any way under compliant conditions, it needs to be done. It can't be an issue of convenience. If a hospital with a non-24/7 pharmacy has a patient who needs an intramuscular (IM) dose of methotrexate prior to the pharmacy re-opening, the on-call pharmacist should go to the hospital to prepare the dose. Centers for Medicare & Medicaid Services (CMS)[10] and accreditation organizations require an on-call pharmacist, and this would be an urgent patient situation where someone needs to be called in. Patients requiring BCG or mitomycin are generally scheduled surgical cases so usually can be prepared in proper facilities when coordinated with the procedural area and pharmacies. In many cases, these procedural areas mix HDs only because "it's always been done that way." Now is the time to speak with the managers in those areas and include them in your educational efforts about the occupational health risks of exposure to HDs. <800> requires that the organization develop standard operating procedures based on the risk of exposure; this is a significant risk and needs to be addressed.

EXHIBIT 15-2 Negative Pressure Technique

Stringent aseptic technique, described by Wilson and Solimando[*] in 1981, remains the foundation of any procedure involving the use of needles and syringes in manipulating sterile dosage forms of HDs. This technique, when performed accurately, minimizes the escape of drug from vials and ampules. Needleless devices have been developed to reduce the risk of blood-borne pathogen exposure to healthcare workers. None of these devices has been tested for reduction of drug escape resulting in residue and surface contamination. The appropriateness of these devices in the safe handling of HDs is unproven. CSTDs, cleared by the FDA under ONB, may provide a solution to syringe and needle compounding of HDs.

Reconstituting HDs in vials. In reconstituting HDs in vials, it is critical to avoid pressurizing the contents of the vial that may cause the drug to spray out around the needle, or through a needle hole or a loose seal, aerosolizing the drug into the compounding area of the Class II BSC or CACI. Pressurization can be avoided by creating a slight negative pressure in the vial. Too much negative pressure, however, can cause leakage from the needle when it is withdrawn from the vial. The safe handling of HD solutions in vials or ampules requires the use of a syringe that is no more than three-quarters (75%) full when filled with the solution. This minimizes the risk of the plunger separating from the syringe barrel. Once the diluent is drawn up, the needle is inserted into the vial and the plunger is pulled back (to create a slight negative pressure inside the vial) so that air is drawn into the syringe. Small amounts of diluent should be transferred slowly as equal volumes of air are removed. The needle should be kept in the vial, and the contents should be swirled carefully until dissolved. With the vial inverted, the proper amount of drug solution should be gradually withdrawn while equal volumes of air are exchanged for solution. The exact volume needed must be measured while the needle is in the vial, and any excess drug should remain in the vial. With the vial in the upright position, a small amount of air should be drawn through the needle and just to the hub of the syringe. No additional air may be drawn into the syringe or that air will require removal prior to measuring or administering the dose. This step would create an opportunity for expelling drug or contaminated air into the environment. The hub should be clear before the needle is removed.

Transferring HD to IV bag. If an HD is transferred to an IV bag, care must be taken to puncture only the septum of the injection port and avoid puncturing the sides of the port or the bag. After the drug solution is injected into the IV bag, the IV port, container, and set (if attached by pharmacy in the Class II BSC or CACI) should be wiped with moist gauze to decontaminate the surfaces. The final preparation should be labeled, including an auxiliary warning, and the injection port covered with a protective shield. Using clean gloves, place the final container into a sealable bag to contain any leakage.[24,32]

Withdrawing HDs from ampuls. To withdraw HDs from an ampul, the neck or top portion should be gently tapped.[109] After the neck is wiped with sterile 70% IPA, a 5-micron filter needle or straw should be attached to a syringe that is large enough that it will be not more than three-quarters (75%) full when holding the drug. Then the fluid should be drawn through the filter needle or straw and cleared from the needle and hub. After this, the needle or straw is exchanged for a needle of similar gauge and length, being careful to dispose of the now HD-contaminated needle or straw. Any air and excess drug should be injected into a sterile vial (leaving the desired volume in the syringe). Aerosols should be avoided. The HD may then be transferred to an IV bag or bottle. If the dose is to be dispensed in the syringe, the plunger should be drawn back to clear fluid from the needle and hub. The needle should be replaced with a locking cap, and the syringe should be

EXHIBIT 15-2 Negative Pressure Technique (cont'd)

wiped with moistened gauze for surface decontamination and labeled. While this technique usually requires more time than compounding with ancillary devices, once mastered, it provides protection to the user even in the absence of other supplemental devices.

*Wilson JP, Solimando DA. Aseptic technique as a safety precaution in the preparation of antineoplastic agents. *Hosp Pharm.* 1981;15:575–81.

BSC: biological safety cabinet; CACI: compounding aseptic containment isolator; CSTD: closed system drug-transfer device; FDA: Food and Drug Administration; HD: hazardous drug; IPA: isopropyl alcohol; IV: intravenous; ONB: FDA product code specifically for a closed antineoplastic and HD reconstitution and transfer system

Source: Reprinted and revised with permission from Power LA, Hazardous drugs as compounded sterile preparations. In: Buchanan CE, Schneider PJ, eds., *Compounding Sterile Preparations,* 3rd ed. Bethesda, MD: ASHP; 2009.

BEYOND-USE DATES 16

16.1 Why is there no BUD information in USP <800>?

USP <800> does not include general compounding information. Beyond-use date (BUD) information can be found in USP <795> for nonsterile compounding and USP <797> for sterile compounding.

16.2 How will a 12-hour BUD work if the drug needs to run longer than that?

BUDs are different from "hang time" of the infusion. The BUD deals with compounding and storage time; it ends when administration of the drug begins. As long as the drug is stable in the container and started prior to 12 hours from the start of compounding, it can run for the time necessary.

16.3 We have a C-SCA and prepare HD pumps for home care patients. The infusion is started within 12 hours of being compounded, but it runs for 144 hours. Is this OK?

Yes. BUDs are defined in USP <795> for nonsterile compounds and in USP <797> for sterile compounds. The BUD deals with compounding and storage time; it ends when administration of the drug begins. As long as the drug is stable in the container and started prior to 12 hours from the start of compounding, it can run for the time necessary.

16.4 Is the maximum BUD for nonsterile compounding described in USP <795>? I don't understand why this isn't included in USP <800>.

USP <800> supplements the compounding requirements of USP <795> for nonsterile compounding and USP <797> for sterile compounding. You need to use the information concerning BUDs in those chapters. Each of the chapters defines the way BUDs are assigned, and they are different processes for the two types of compounds (nonsterile and sterile).

PACKAGING 17

(See Sections 11 and 12 in <800>.)

<800> allows the entity to perform an Assessment of Risk to evaluate exempting specific dosage forms of HDs from the containment strategies and/or work practices. Antineoplastics that require only counting or packaging, non-antineoplastic agents, and reproductive hazards may be considered for the entity's Assessment of Risk if alternative containment strategies and/or work practices are identified and implemented.

17.1 Is unit dosing of antineoplastics considered compounding, and does it have to be performed in a controlled environment?

Pre-packaging of antineoplastics isn't compounding, but it *is* covered under <800> since it is handling a hazardous drug (HD). If you include this in your Assessment of Risk, you may exempt dosage forms of antineoplastics that require only counting or packaging. Oral tablets could be considered for this. However, if you have the appropriate facilities for compounding HDs, why not use them to protect personnel during pre-packaging, too?

This is a two-step issue:
(1) The pharmacy staff would have a higher level of risk, since they need to directly handle the HDs. (2) Once they are packaged, the risk of handling the finished dosage form is reduced. Consider using your containment device (containment ventilated enclosure [CVE], biological safety cabinet [BSC], or compounding aseptic containment isolator [CACI]) as the location where your oral antineoplastics are packaged. If using a BSC or CACI in your negative pressure sterile compounding area, you would need to use the same restrictions as you would for nonsterile compounding: do this only while no sterile compounding is occurring, and decontaminate, clean, and disinfect the surfaces following completion of the pre-packaging. In any case, consider restricting specific counting trays and spatulas for HDs you package, and include specific instructions in your procedures for decontamination and cleaning the equipment.

17.2 Is it OK to use a packaging machine to unit dose HDs?

Solid oral antineoplastics must not be placed in packaging or counting devices because that process could create powders, which would contaminate the system. Use a manual unit-dose system for oral antineoplastic agents, and consider using your containment device (CVE, BSC, or CACI) in which to do the packaging. For non-antineoplastic and reproductive hazards in solid oral formulations, you can address alternative containment strategies in your Assessment of Risk. For example, you might dedicate specific equipment for this, decide to use a manual system, or perform the pre-packaging in your containment device.

17.3 Which oral dosage forms of HDs don't require counting in negative rooms?

This depends on your Assessment of Risk. If you determine alternative containment strategies, you could exempt solid oral dosage forms of non-antineoplastics and/or reproductive hazards from this requirement.

17.4 Even though <800> allows antineoplastics in final forms that require only counting or packaging, why wouldn't I use a powder hood or BSC to pre-package them?

If you have the proper facility, use your powder hood or BSC to limit risk to personnel who are pre-packaging or counting antineoplastics.

17.5 What precautions are needed for crushing tablets or opening capsules of HDs?

This is manipulation of a HD. Pharmacy should be packaging these dosage forms, so nursing or other staff do not have to manipulate the drug in an area without the controls of a negative primary engineering control (PEC) or negative room. Additionally, providing ready-to-use dosage forms is expected by the Centers for Medicare & Medicaid Services (CMS) and accreditation organizations.

17.6 Our obstetric department uses misoprostol in 25-mcg tablets. They are available only in 100-mcg tablets. How can we best comply with their needs?

Misoprostol is on Table 3 (reproductive hazards) in the National Institute for Occupational Safety and Health (NIOSH) list of HDs.[5] All containment strategies in <800> are required unless you consider this in your Assessment of Risk.

If you include it in your Assessment of Risk, you could consider some of these approaches:
- Define restrictions concerning who may package the 25-mcg doses, based on the reason misoprostol is on the list.
- Dedicate a specific tablet splitter only for misoprostol use.
- Develop a method to place the quarter-tablets in a consistent packaging system (e.g., a manual unit-dose bubble).
- Label the bag with whatever caution is required by your Assessment of Risk.
- Place the doses in a lidded container in the automated dispensing cabinet (ADC) with a warning on the lid.

17.7 Do patient-specific doses of antineoplastic oral solution HDs need to be drawn up in a negative pressure room? How about non-antineoplastic HD oral solutions?

This is manipulation of a HD, so containment strategies are necessary. <800> permits use of the BSC or CACI in your sterile negative pressure compounding room for occasional nonsterile use, as long as the stipulations listed in <800> are followed. If you do this routinely, you need to have the proper equipment for nonsterile HD compounding/repackaging.

17.8 Is it OK to use a packaging machine for HDs that aren't antineoplastic?

For agents that are non-antineoplastic or reproductive hazards only, you could consider them in your Assessment of Risk. Evaluate if the dosage forms could break, which would contaminate your equipment.

17.9 How are hospitals managing warfarin administration if it requires cutting/splitting of tablets?

Warfarin is on Table 3 (reproductive hazards) in the NIOSH list of HDs.[5] All containment strategies in <800> are required unless you consider this in your Assessment of Risk.

If you include it in your Assessment of Risk, you could consider some of these approaches:
- Define restrictions concerning who may package the half-tablets, based on the reason warfarin is on the list.
- Dedicate a specific tablet splitter only for warfarin use.
- Develop a method to place the half-tablets in a consistent packaging system (e.g., a manual unit-dose bubble).
- Label the bag with whatever caution is required by your Assessment of Risk.

<800> allows nursing to split one dose of a HD using appropriate personal protective equipment (PPE) (as defined in your policy) and containing the drug in a plastic pouch. However, there are other issues beyond <800> here. CMS and hospital accreditation organizations expect pharmacy to provide ready-to-use dosage forms. For all these reasons, splitting tablets of HDs should be done by pharmacy under proper conditions.

17.10 Who crushes tablets for nasogastric tube administration—pharmacy or nursing?

This is manipulation of a HD, so it needs to be done under proper conditions. <800> allows nursing to crush one dose of a HD using appropriate PPE (as defined in your policy) and containing the drug in a plastic pouch. However, there are other issues beyond <800> here. CMS and hospital accreditation organizations expect pharmacy to provide ready-to-use dosage forms. For all these reasons, crushing tablets of HDs should be done by pharmacy under proper conditions whenever possible.

17.11 What precautions should be taken when unit-dosing liquids are on the HD list?

Liquid oral antineoplastics must be packaged under <800>-compliant conditions—in a C-PEC with full garb. For HDs that are non-antineoplastic or reproductive hazards, you could consider them in your Assessment of Risk.

17.12 If pharmacy unit doses a HD, does that mean it's a final dosage form?

Although really a semantic difference, consider it a finished dosage form since a final dosage form is related to a U.S. Food and Drug Administration (FDA) product.

You need to consider a phased approach in your Assessment of Risk: If a drug is purchased in a bulk bottle (as a final dosage form from a conventional manufacturer), the risk to pharmacy personnel is different (since they need to package it) than it is to nursing (who receives it as a ready-to-use unit dose). You would have to consider the different safety needs. For example, even though azathioprine is on the non-antineoplastic table of the NIOSH list of HDs,[5] you might treat it with full antineoplastic precautions in the pharmacy because it's received in a bulk bottle. You might package it in your BSC with full garb, using the process listed in USP <800> for occasional nonsterile compounding in a sterile compounding suite. However, once it is packaged, you might require only one pair of chemo gloves when nursing administers the agent.

17.13 After I have compounded or packaged nonsterile antineoplastic agents into the finished dosage form, how do I need to store them prior to dispensing or patient pick-up?

You can define this in your Assessment of Risk. If you have alternative containment strategies (e.g., placing each dispensing unit in a plastic overwrap), you may be able to store them with your other stock. Consider using a designated bin in which to store these finished containers to alert staff that they are hazardous. They do not need to be labeled as hazardous for the patient labeling unless manufacturer information or your policy requires you to do so.

17.14 USP <800> says that when you make a non-HD in a chemo hood, you have to label it with PPE handling precautions. Where are the precautions listed? Are they in the Safety Data Sheet, Department of Transportation information, or somewhere else?

You need to define them in your policies. The point is to alert a healthcare worker that the preparation may be contaminated with HDs (because you compounded it in your HD PEC).

DISPENSING HAZARDOUS DRUGS 18

18.1 Do I need a separate counting tray for each different HD?

Not unless that is required by your Assessment of Risk. However, you should dedicate specific equipment (e.g., counting trays, spatulas, mortar and pestles) for use with hazardous drugs (HDs). The equipment needs to be decontaminated after each use.

See Section 21, Decontamination and Cleaning, for further information.

18.1 DISPENSING FINISHED DOSAGE FORMS TO PATIENT CARE UNITS

18.1-1 What precautions need to be taken for chemo bags between the pharmacy, and where will they be administered?

Your policy needs to define the specific details. For example, you should have a detailed policy and practice concerning packaging of the HD compounded sterile preparation (CSP) as it is removed from the biological safety cabinet (BSC) or compounding aseptic containment isolator (CACI); this should include assurance that the outer chemo bag is free from contamination. If they need to be transported to an area separate from where they are mixed, they must be in an impervious container. The personnel who transport the HD CSPs need to have documented competence to do so, must wear personal protective equipment (PPE) as defined by your policy, and need to know what to do in case of a spill.

If the agents have to be transported to a different campus of your health system, additional training of transport personnel and compliance with Department of Transportation regulations also must be included.

18.1-2 Is it OK to store HDs in ADCs?

This depends on your Assessment of Risk. Because only final or finished dosage forms would be stored in an automated dispensing cabinet (ADC), you could establish containment practices that provide an additional layer of safety. You would probably want to treat antineoplastic agents differently from most of the non-antineoplastics and reproductive hazards. You might determine that your current unit-dose packaging is adequate containment for those drugs on the National Institute for Occupational Safety and Health (NIOSH) lists of non-antineoplastics and reproductive hazards. Since few antineoplastics are likely to be placed in an ADC, you could package them in an additional sealable bag to further contain any potential contamination.

18.1-3 Is it OK to deliver HDs in pneumatic tubes?

USP <800> specifically prohibits placement of antineoplastics or any liquid HDs in pneumatic tubes because of the potential for breakage and contamination.

18.2 DISPENSING FINISHED DOSAGE FORMS TO AMBULATORY PATIENTS

18.2-1 What precautions need to be taken for an oral chemo dispensed and waiting for patient pick-up?

That depends on your Assessment of Risk. USP <800> has no requirement to label ambulatory prescriptions as hazardous. There may be manufacturer's requirements that must be followed. Consider placement in a separate area and/or additional packaging around the container, which would provide an additional safety level.

18.2-2 Do I need to decontaminate a nonsterile HD preparation after I make it?

Yes, and your policy needs to define the specific details. For example, you should have a detailed policy and practice concerning packaging of the HD preparation as it is removed from the primary engineering control (PEC); this needs to include assurance that the outside of the container is free from contamination. If it needs to be transported to an area separate from where it is mixed, it must be in an impervious container. The personnel who transport the HD compounded preparations need to have documented competence to do so, must wear PPE as defined by your policy, and must know what to do in case of a spill.

If the agents have to be transported to a different campus of your health system, additional training of transport personnel and compliance with Department of Transportation regulations also must be included.

18.2-3 The NIOSH list states that single gloves should be worn with administration from unit-dose packages. How does this impact community pharmacies where pharmacists and technicians have the potential to touch these final dosage forms during dispensing?

No one other than the patient should touch any drug. Your Assessment of Risk and policies should require use of PPE (e.g., a single pair of chemo gloves) when counting and packaging antineoplastics. The counting tray, spatula, and any other equipment or supplies used should be decontaminated after each use if the items are reusable.

See Section 21, Decontamination and Cleaning, for further information.

TRANSPORTING HAZARDOUS DRUGS 19

(See Section 11 in <800>.)

APIs of any HD and antineoplastics (except those that require only counting or packaging) must comply with all containment listed in <800>. <800> allows the entity to perform an Assessment of Risk to evaluate exempting specific dosage forms of HDs from the containment strategies and/or work practices. Antineoplastics that require only counting or packaging, non-antineoplastic agents, and reproductive hazards may be considered for the entity's Assessment of Risk if alternative containment strategies and/or work practices are identified and implemented.

19.1 Why can't pneumatic tubes be used for transporting HDs?

USP <800> does not allow use of pneumatic tubes for transport of any antineoplastics or any liquid hazardous drugs (HDs) because a breakage would contaminate the entire tube system.

19.2 Can HDs be transported in tubes, robots, patient carts, etc.?

Liquid HDs and any antineoplastic HD cannot be transported in pneumatic tubes because a breakage or leakage would contaminate the entire tube system. Use your Assessment of Risk to determine if the other methods of transport are acceptable.

19.3 Can volunteers transport finished chemo to our oncology center?

This is a problematic practice. Any personnel—employees, volunteers, or students—must have the same competencies to perform tasks. This means that they must complete the health system's Occupational Safety and Health Administration (OSHA) training as well as your HD training and competencies. This includes use of personal protective equipment (PPE) and spill management. Most organizations will not want to place their volunteers in this situation. Check with your Risk Management department to see if they would support this practice. Some state boards of pharmacy have additional requirements concerning personnel permitted to handle medications.

ADMINISTERING HAZARDOUS DRUGS 20

(See Section 14 in <800>.)

APIs of any HD and antineoplastics (except those that require only counting or packaging) must comply with all containment listed in <800>, which allows the entity to perform an Assessment of Risk to evaluate exempting specific dosage forms of HDs from the containment strategies and/or work practices. Antineoplastics that require only counting or packaging, non-antineoplastic agents, and reproductive hazards may be considered for the entity's Assessment of Risk if alternative containment strategies and/or work practices are identified and implemented.

20.1 What PPE is required for administration of parenteral HDs?

Two pairs of chemotherapy gloves and a gown shown to resist permeability by hazardous drugs (HDs) are required for administration of parenteral antineoplastic agents. The organization's policy needs to define personal protective equipment (PPE) for other HDs. Some organizations require gowns to be worn for any hazardous medication if they are liquid, manipulated on the patient care unit (e.g., crushing tablets or opening capsules), or inhaled. Additionally, some organizations require gowns to be worn for men and women who are trying to conceive, women who are pregnant, and women who are breast-feeding.

20.2 Is PPE (other than gloves) required for the administration of oral HDs?

This needs to be part of your policy and procedure and included in your Assessment of Risk.

20.3 Is there a list of recommended PPE to wear based on the dosage form administered?

Yes. The National Institute for Occupational Safety and Health (NIOSH) list of HDs[5] has a list of recommended PPE based on the dosage form administered and the manipulation required to administer that dose.

20.4 If nurses have to wear gloves for administration of HDs, do they need to change the gloves between patients?

Of course. They would not use a single pair of gloves for multiple patients.

20.5 Can a nurse crush a HD tablet at the bedside?

USP <800> allows a nurse to crush a single dose if necessary, provided they don appropriate PPE (as defined by your policy) and use a plastic pouch to contain any particles. However, if possible, pharmacy should do this under the proper containment conditions and provide a ready-to-administer form to the nurse.

20.6 What does <800> means by a *plastic pouch* to contain particles?

Plastic pouches are commercially available from pharmacy suppliers. They are individual pouches that can be used with a tablet crusher to contain any particles. The pouch is sturdy enough to withstand crushing and can be used as the container to administer the drug or place the drug in another vehicle (e.g., applesauce) for administration.

20.7 What PPE should a nurse wear when crushing HDs?

That needs to be defined in your Assessment of Risk. USP <800>[8] requires appropriate PPE and use of a plastic pouch. The appendix of the 2016 NIOSH list of HDs[8] recommends use of a gown, double gloves, and respiratory protection.

20.8 Our Emergency Department nurses might administer IM methotrexate at night when the pharmacy is closed. Do they need to take any precautions when they prepare the dose?

Nursing should *not* be doing this without the proper facilities; pharmacy should come in to prepare that dose in the proper facilities.

20.9 Why do nurses need to use a CSTD when administering chemo?

Pharmacy has robust engineering controls—hoods and negative pressure rooms—that protect the compounder. Without closed system drug-transfer devices (CSTDs), nurses have no protection other than PPE. The CSTD provides protection to personnel and the environment while they are administering antineoplastic agents.

20.10 What precautions must be made for administering oral chemotherapy through a feeding tube? There are issues in mixing the doses administered to the patient, but there are no CSTDs for this process.

Many of the oral oncology agents have no stability information available, so pre-packaging and/or pre-mixing them is often not supported. Nursing may need to crush the tablet or open the capsule at the bedside and immediately administer the agent through a tube. Of course, check with the manufacturer for information. Evaluate this in your Assessment of Risk and include the specific details (e.g., PPE, procedure) to be used. USP <800> requires use of a CSTD to administer a drug when the dosage form allows; because no such CSTD is available at this time, it does not need to be included in your procedure.

20.11 What happens when a stat oxytocin drip is needed?

Oxytocin is listed on Table 3 (reproductive hazards) of the NIOSH list of HDs.[5] It is a *situational hazard* to women in the third trimester of pregnancy. It can be handled in your Assessment of Risk, but be sure to include protection from staff who are in their third trimester of pregnancy; they should not be mixing the drug. *This particular situation is much easier to solve than some other drugs:* provide premixed, standardized solutions to your obstetric department. Be sure Anesthesia is involved in the policy and procedure development because they are usually the personnel who would mix the drug. Other than a rare need for an intramuscular (IM) dose (which should also be part of your Assessment of Risk), there is no need for anyone to prepare this drug on the patient care unit.

20.12 What precautions must be in place for the nursing staff who administer HDs to patients in an outpatient infusion setting?

All personnel who come in contact with HDs need to be trained and their competency assessed. This includes wearing appropriate PPE, use of CSTDs, and other requirements of <800>.

20.13 Does a non-antineoplastic drug like premixed oxytocin require a CSTD?

That depends on your Assessment of Risk. Most organizations will limit use of CSTDs to antineoplastics, but that decision is up to you.

20.14 Where can I find nursing competencies?

The Compounding Hazardous Drugs chapter in *Competence Assessment Tools for Health-System Pharmacies*[12] (see **Appendix**) and Oncology Nursing Society's *Safe Handling of Hazardous Drugs*[11] have information that can be developed into nursing-specific competencies.

DECONTAMINATION AND CLEANING 21

(See Section 15 in <800>.)

APIs of any HD and antineoplastics (except those that require only counting or packaging) must comply with all containment listed in <800>, which allows the entity to perform an Assessment of Risk to evaluate exempting specific dosage forms of HDs from the containment strategies and/or work practices. Antineoplastics that require only counting or packaging, non-antineoplastic agents, and reproductive hazards may be considered for the entity's Assessment of Risk.

21.1 What is the difference between cleaning and decontamination?

There are several steps in this process:
- Deactivation and decontamination, which makes a compound inactive and removes it by transferring the residue to a disposable material (e.g., a low-lint wipe).
- Cleaning removes contaminants by use of a germicidal detergent.
- Disinfection inhibits or destroys microorganisms.

21.2 How is cleaning a chemo hood different from what's done for the regular hood?

Areas—hoods and rooms—used for handling hazardous drugs (HDs) need to be decontaminated prior to cleaning. Where surfaces used for handling non-HDs need to be cleaned and, if used for sterile compounding, disinfected, surfaces used for handling HDs have the additional preliminary step of deactivating the HD and decontaminating the surfaces. Cleaning and disinfection follows.

21.3 Do I need to wear PPE when cleaning?

Yes. In addition to the head, hair, shoe covers, gowns, and gloves, you need to wear eye protection when splashing is possible (e.g., cleaning ceilings, walls) and respiratory protection when necessary.

21.4 Is it OK for Environmental Services to clean the floors while we are compounding?

No. You cannot compound while cleaning is occurring.

21.5 What agents deactivate HDs?

Few drugs have specific deactivators. Traditionally, bleach has been used for this purpose. If the drug has a specific deactivator listed in the product labeling, use it after manipulating that drug.

21.6 What agents decontaminate HD areas?

Use a properly diluted (if required) Environmental Protection Agency (EPA)-approved oxidizing agent intended for use with HDs. Traditionally, bleach has been used in a 2% concentration, followed by sodium thiosulfate to neutralize the bleach. (Bleach left on stainless steel surfaces will corrode the surface, causing pitting and rust.) There are now commercially available agents for this purpose.

21.7 What agents clean HD areas?

Germicidal detergents are the cleaning agents for sterile compounding as defined in USP <797> and are appropriate for nonsterile areas, too. Once decontamination has been done, the cleaning and disinfection steps are the same as with non-hazardous compounding.

21.8 What agents disinfect HD areas?

Disinfecting agents for sterile compounding are defined in USP <797> and are appropriate for nonsterile areas, too. Alcohol (sterile alcohol for sterile compounding) is the predominant agent. Once decontamination has been done, the cleaning and disinfection steps are the same as with non-hazardous compounding.

21.9 Is alcohol sufficient to decontaminate and clean the HD areas?

No. Alcohol is neither a decontaminating agent nor a cleaner. Alcohol is a disinfectant and is useful only in the final step after deactivation, decontaminating, and cleaning has occurred.

21.10 Who should clean the BSC and CACI?

Only compounding personnel may decontaminate, clean, and disinfect the primary engineering controls (PECs).

21.11 Who should clean the SECs?

Either compounding personnel or Environmental Services personnel can decontaminate, clean, and disinfect the anteroom, buffer room, or containment segregated compounding area (C-SCA). Training and documented competence is required. In any case, all compounding personnel should be competent in this task in case Environmental Services is not available.

21.12 Are there specific cleaning guidelines under USP <800>?

USP <800> contains a section on Deactivation, Decontamination, Cleaning, and Disinfection. There is more detail in USP <797>. (See both the current 2008 version of USP <797>[18] and the proposed revision of USP <797>.[22])

21.13 Is there a single process I can use to deactivate all HDs?

No. Unfortunately, the information about deactivation is limited. That is why decontamination (removal of the contamination) is so important.

21.14 What concentration of bleach should I use?

If you use bleach to deactivate and decontaminate HD surfaces, use about a 2% concentration. Most commercial bleach is about 5.25%, so one part bleach to two parts water is an appropriate dilution. Be sure to remove the bleach from stainless steel surfaces. Traditionally, sodium thiosulfate has been used; since the next step in the process is cleaning the area, use of the cleaner is sufficient to remove the bleach.

21.15 How do I know I am using the correct dilutions of decontamination and cleaning solutions?

Read the manufacturer's instructions. Ready-to-use solutions are the most convenient because they do not require dilution. Be sure that the solutions remain in contact with the surface for the appropriate contact time; that information will be in the manufacturer's instructions.

21.16 Do I need to clean the whole hood between mixing different chemo preps?

Not necessarily. USP <800> requires that the work surface of the C-PEC must be decontaminated between compounding of different HDs. The entire C-PEC must be decontaminated, cleaned, and disinfected at least daily when it is used, any time a spill occurs, before and after certification, any time voluntary interruption occurs, and if it is moved. The work tray under the biological safety cabinet (BSC) or compounding aseptic containment isolator (CACI) needs to be decontaminated, cleaned, and disinfected at least monthly.

21.17 What should I use to decontaminate the chemo hood between chemo preps?

Consider using wipes pre-saturated with a decontaminating agent.

21.18 Why shouldn't I use a spray bottle of alcohol?

No agents should be sprayed in a HD area. Spraying can aerosolize and spread contamination.

21.19 What should I use to disinfect the chemo hood between preparations?

Consider using wipes pre-saturated with alcohol. The alcohol must be sterile when compounding sterile preparations.

21.20 How do I decontaminate the floor?

At least once a week, supplement or substitute use of a decontaminating agent with your daily germicidal detergent cleaning.

21.21 How often should I use sterile alcohol to clean the floor?

Alcohol is not a cleaner; it is a disinfecting agent. There is no value in using alcohol or sterile alcohol for this purpose.

21.22 Are specific cleaning supplies required by USP <800>?

USP <797> and USP <800> provide guidance for types of products and devices (e.g., mops), but it is up to you to develop your policies and procedures.

21.23 Are reusable mops acceptable to use?

They are not prohibited, but consider the process you use. Standardizing on disposable mop heads removes the concern of spreading contamination from the HD areas as well as the concern of bringing microbial contamination into the compounding areas.

21.24 What is the best way to monitor that cleaning has been done?

Routine cleaning of the C-PEC throughout the compounding day should be a part of your practice. The Designated Person should monitor that this is being done. Some states require documentation throughout the day. If this is required, be sure that papers and writing implements do not compromise the microbial burden of the room. Daily and monthly cleaning should be documented.

21.25 What do I do about a rusty hood?

The hood probably needs to be replaced. Rust is unacceptable in a sterile compounding area.

21.26 How can I tell if we are removing the contaminants?

You can check by doing wipe sampling of the surfaces.

See Section 22, Environmental Monitoring.

ENVIRONMENTAL MONITORING 22

(See Sections 6 and 17 in <800>.)

APIs of any HD and antineoplastics (except those that require only counting or packaging) must comply with all containment listed in <800>, which allows the entity to perform an Assessment of Risk to evaluate exempting specific dosage forms of HDs from the containment strategies and/or work practices. Antineoplastics that require only counting or packaging, non-antineoplastic agents, and reproductive hazards may be considered for the entity's Assessment of Risk if alternative containment strategies and/or work practices are identified and implemented.

22.1 What types of quality assurance and quality control activities are required or recommended in USP <800>?

USP <795> (for nonsterile compounding) and USP <797> (for sterile compounding) contain information on general compounding quality control and quality assurance expectations. The environmental monitoring in USP <797> deals with monitoring of microbial (bacterial and fungal) contamination; this is still required for compounding sterile hazardous drug (HD) preparations.

In addition, USP <800> recommends—but does not require—environmental monitoring for HD contamination. This type of environmental monitoring is accomplished by taking surface wipe samples of areas where HDs are handled.

22.2 USP <795> doesn't include a requirement for microbial monitoring for nonsterile compounding areas. Should this be considered?

It is not required but should be considered. If there is a contamination of the containment ventilated enclosure (CVE) or nonsterile compounding room, the quality of the nonsterile compound will be affected.

22.3 Is surface sampling the only quality point that needs to be considered?

No.

USP <795>,[21] <797>,[18] <800>,[8] and the other USP general chapters that support compounding activities require or recommend other quality elements, including:

- Personnel training
- Personnel monitoring
- Microbial environmental monitoring
- Certification of the primary engineering controls (PECs) and secondary engineering controls (SECs)
- Documentation

22.4 Are wipe samples required?

No, but they are recommended.

22.5 Are there different requirements if we are using an isolator instead of a BSC?

USP <800> does not differentiate based on the type of C-PEC used. The requirements and recommendations are the same.

22.6 How often should wipe samples be collected?

USP <800> recommends—but does not require—collection of benchmark samples and then repeated samples at least every 6 months to verify that HDs are contained.

22.7 Where should wipe samples be collected?

Suggested areas include inside the biological safety cabinet (BSC) or compounding aseptic containment isolator (CACI), pass-through chambers, surfaces near the BSC or CACI, the floor underneath the front of the C-PEC, areas immediately outside the negative pressure room, and areas where patients are administered antineoplastics.

22.8 Are we likely to find contamination?

Yes. You will likely find measurable levels of the antineoplastics that you handle.

22.9 What drugs are commonly assayed?

Common drugs that most companies evaluate are cyclophosphamide, ifosfamide, methotrexate, fluorouracil, and platinum-based agents. Detection of other agents may be available from the companies.

22.10 How many surface samples are usually taken?

Most companies provide six wipes with instructions for use. The wipes are returned to the company for analysis, and you receive a report with the results.

22.11 What action do we need to take if antineoplastic contamination is found? How can we get the level to zero?

It is unlikely that repeat sampling will reveal zero contamination, but changes in your practice should reduce the levels.

Practice changes to consider include: re-training personnel; changes in work practices; comprehensive decontamination, cleaning, and disinfecting HD areas; and improving engineering controls.

22.12 What is the responsibility of the *designated person* regarding surface sampling results?

The *designated person* needs to identify, document, and implement processes to improve the results.

22.13 What are the acceptable limits for the results of HD surface contamination?

No acceptable limits are currently defined. Contamination in any amount shows that a lack of containment has occurred. This needs to be addressed with practice changes.

22.14 Once contamination is found on wipe samples and the issue is addressed, should we expect the next levels to show zero contamination?

That is unlikely, but you should see a decrease in the level if your remediation efforts have been effective.

22.15 Why is surface sampling only *recommended* and *not required*?

This is an emerging area of quality control. There are no certifying agencies for vendors of wipe sample kits. There are no standards for acceptable limits for HD surface contamination. However, it is an important element of quality control and needs to be considered as part of a safe workplace control.

HAZARDOUS WASTE 23

(See Section 11 in <800>.)

USP <800> deals with HDs that are an occupational exposure risk. This is different from EPA hazardous materials—some of which are drugs—that are hazards to the environment.

23.1 Does it seem like the section about disposal got the short end of the stick? It just says "all applicable federal, state, and local regulations."[8] Disposition of hazardous components within the healthcare setting seems to me to be just as important as the other areas listed in the chapter.

It is important although a different issue from the intent of <800>, which deals with hazardous drugs (HDs) that are hazardous to healthcare personnel. The issue of disposal of hazardous materials is an Environmental Protection Agency (EPA) issue. Those regulations differ by state and region. They are beyond the scope of <800>.

23.2 Is proper disposal of HDs part of a compounder's responsibilities under USP <800>?

Yes. USP <800> requires compliance with all applicable federal, state, and local regulations.

23.3 Who can provide the information our health system needs to know about disposal of HDs and the federal and state requirements?

The health system's waste hauler is the best source for this information.

23.4 Does pharmacy need to control the handling of hazardous materials for the health system?

No, not unless that is part of your specific responsibility. HDs are just a portion of the hazardous materials that a health system needs to control. Be sure that your direct report and facilities personnel are aware of the distinction between National Institute for Occupational Safety and Health (NIOSH) HDs (which are hazardous to healthcare personnel) and EPA hazardous materials (which are hazardous to the environment), and include many more substances than drugs.

SPILLS 24

(See Section 16 in <800>.)

APIs of any HD and antineoplastics (except those that require only counting or packaging) must comply with all containment listed in <800>, which allows the entity to perform an Assessment of Risk to evaluate exempting specific dosage forms of HDs from the containment strategies and/or work practices. Antineoplastics that require only counting or packaging, non-antineoplastic agents, and reproductive hazards may be considered for the entity's Assessment of Risk if alternative containment strategies and/or work practices are identified and implemented.

24.1 What is a *spill*?

A *spill* occurs any time a hazardous drug (HD) is not contained in its intended container (including a bottle, intravenous bag, syringe, and other containers). A solid, intact dosage form may not be an issue, but a liquid or particulates need to be handled as a spill.

24.2 Are antineoplastic agents the only concern?

Any drug could have some noxious properties. Check in the package insert or Safety Data Sheet (SDS) for details.

24.3 What is a *spill kit*?

A *spill kit* is a type of emergency supply used to clean up a spill. It needs to contain the appropriate supplies, based on the type of drugs and dosage forms handled.

24.4 What spill kit contents does USP <800> require?

There are no specific contents required by USP <800>. You need to design your spill kit to meet your needs.

24.5 Is there a standard spill kit that I can purchase?

Several suppliers market spill kits. If you choose to use them, be sure they contain the supplies you would need in case of a spill.

24.6 Where do spill kits need to be located?

Spill kits need to be available in all locations where HDs are handled.

24.7 What should be in a spill kit?

The spill kit needs to contain supplies to contain and clean up a spill. Appendix H of the *ASHP Guidelines on Handling Hazardous Drugs*[3] contains a list of suggested components.

The spill kit should include items such as
- Personal protective equipment (PPE)
- Spill pads and towels
- Rigid containers for collection of spill contents and cleanup materials
- Disposable scoop

24.8 How big a spill can a spill kit handle?

Commercially available spill kits are designed for small spills. A single spill kit will not likely be able to handle a large spill.

24.9 What resources can I use to develop a policy concerning spill cleanup?

Appendix I of the *ASHP Guidelines on Handling Hazardous Drugs*[3] contains recommendations for spill cleanup procedures.

24.10 Who should clean up a spill?

You need to determine that in your policy. The person who first notices the spill needs to contain it to the extent possible, then either continue the cleanup or call for help. USP <800> requires availability of personnel qualified to clean up a spill anytime and anyplace HDs are handled in healthcare settings. Consider developing a Spill Response Team at your organization.

24.11 If a facility contracts Hazmat for all hazardous spills, do infusion staff still need to be trained in HD spill cleanup, and are spill kits required in cleanrooms?

Spill kits need to be in all areas where HDs are handled. Spill management should be a competency that is documented for all personnel who handle HDs. Not all personnel need to be expected to handle all situations, but they need to know how to contain a spill, who to call, where the spill kit and other supplies are located, and other components of the organization's procedure. Personnel who could respond to a spill need to be available at all times when HDs are compounded and administered. Your policy and procedure should include response to small versus large spills. Infusion staff are the front line of this issue, so they should know how to handle a spill based on your organization's policy.

24.12 What is the best way to test our policy and procedure?

Consider having a spill drill. Involve pharmacy, infusion nursing, and environmental services. This is a good way to evaluate competency and is likely to show you what additional supplies you must have available to handle a spill.

WHAT DO I DO NOW? 25

25.1 I'm overwhelmed with this information. Where do I start?

- Read USP <800>.
- Read the National Institute for Occupational Safety and Health (NIOSH) list of hazardous drugs (HDs) and determine the HDs (and the particular dosage forms) that you handle.
- Perform a gap analysis.
- Assign a Designated Person and provide needed resources (e.g., educational programs).
- Examine your certification report, discuss non-compliant issues with your certifier, and take steps to become compliant. Identify the facility issues you need to improve and obtain administrative approval for any renovations needed.
- Work with your Designated Person to ensure personnel training and policy development.
- Ensure your decontamination and cleaning solutions and policies are appropriate.

25.2 Where can I find a gap analysis?

Gap analyses are available at www.hazmedsafety.com and at www.800gaptool.com.

25.3 What can I do to comply with <800> while waiting for capital improvements to my compounding facility to be completed?

Personnel training, policy and procedure development, and evaluating your decontamination and cleaning processes are vital. Stage a spill drill with pharmacy, infusion nursing, and Environmental Services.

25.4 Is there a template Action Plan I could use to start assessing the compliance at my organization?

Exhibit 25-1 is an example of an action plan.

EXHIBIT 25-1 — Action Plan for Compliance with USP <800>

	Element	Assigned To	Completed
List of HDs	Use 2016 NIOSH list		
Assessment of Risk	Determine approach		
Designated Person			
Personnel Training			
PPE	Gloves		
	Gowns		
	Double shoe covers		
Receiving	Training		
	Identify HD packages		
	Assess integrity of packages		
	Spill kit		
Transport	Receiving to storage		
	Completed CSP to units		
Nonsterile Storage and Compounding Room			
Sterile Storage and Compounding Room			
CSTDs			
Cleaning	Deactivate/decontaminate		
	Germicidal detergent		
	Sterile alcohol		
Spill Control	Policy		
	Spill kit contents		
	Spill kit locations		

CSP: compounded sterile preparation; CSTD: closed system drug-transfer device; HD: hazardous drug; NIOSH: National Institute for Occupational Safety and Health; PPE: personal protective equipment

FUTURE EDITIONS

Do you have questions that were not answered? Feel free to submit questions that can be included in the next edition of this publication. Send the questions to publications@ashp.org.

REFERENCES

1. ASHP. ASHP technical assistance bulletin on handling cytotoxic drugs in hospitals. *Am J Hosp Pharm.* 1985;42:131-7.
2. ASHP. ASHP technical assistance bulletin on handling cytotoxic and hazardous drugs. *Am J Hosp Pharm.* 1990;47:1033-49.
3. ASHP. ASHP guidelines on handling hazardous drugs. *Am J Health-Syst Pharm.* 2006;63:1172-93.
4. Centers for Disease Control and Prevention. NIOSH Alert on *Preventing Occupational Exposure to Antineoplastic and Other Hazardous Drugs in Health Care Settings,* 2004. Publication number 2004-165. http://www.cdc.gov/niosh/docs/2004-165/pdfs/2004-165.pdf. Accessed 25 September 2016.
5. NIOSH List of *Antineoplastic and Other Hazardous Drugs in Healthcare Settings,* 2016. Publication number 2016-161. http://www.cdc.gov/niosh/docs/2014-138/pdfs/2016-161/pdf. Accessed 25 September 2016.
6. Occupational Safety and Health Administration. Controlling occupational exposure to hazardous drugs. https://www.osha.gov/SLTC/hazardousdrugs/controlling_occex_hazardousdrugs.html. Accessed 25 September 2016.
7. Occupational exposure to antineoplastics and other hazardous drugs, http://www.cdc.gov/niosh/topics/antineoplastic/default.html. Accessed 25 September 2016.
8. United States Pharmacopeial Convention. General chapter <800> hazardous drugs—handling in healthcare settings. *USP 40–NF 35;* 2017.
9. Centers for Medicare & Medicaid Services, State Operations Manual, Appendix A—Survey Protocol, Regulations and Interpretive Guidelines for Hospitals. https://www.cms.gov/Regulations-and-Guidance/Guidance/Manuals/downloads/som107ap_a_hospitals.pdf. Accessed 25 September 2016.
10. Centers for Disease Control and Prevention. NIOSH Workplace Solutions, *Medical Surveillance for Health Care Workers Exposed to Hazardous Drugs,* 2007. Publication number 2013-103. http://www.cdc.gov/niosh/docs/wp-solutions/2013-103/pdfs/2013-103.pdf. Accessed 19 May 2016.
11. Polovich M. *Safe Handling of Hazardous Drugs,* 2nd ed. Pittsburgh, PA: Oncology Nursing Society; 2011.
12. Murdaugh LB. *Competence Assessment Tools for Health-System Pharmacies,* 5th ed. Bethesda, MD: ASHP; 2015.
13. Centers for Disease Control and Prevention. NIOSH Workplace Solutions, *Personal Protective Equipment for Health Care Workers Who Work with Hazardous Drugs,* 2008. Publication number 2009-106. http://www.cdc.gov/niosh/docs/wp-solutions/2009-106/pdfs/2009-106.pdf. Accessed 25 September 2016.
14. ASTM D6978-05 (2013). Standard Practice for Assessment of Resistance of Medical Gloves to Permeation by Chemotherapy Drugs. West Conshohocken, PA: ASTM International.
15. ASTM F739-99a. Standard Test Method for Resistance of Protective Clothing Materials to Permeation by Liquids or Gases under Conditions of Continuous Contact. West Conshohocken, PA: ASTM International.
16. NSF/ANSI 49-2004. Class II (laminar flow) Biosafety Cabinetry, NSF International. Ann Arbor, MI 48113-0140. www.nsf.org
17. CETA International, Application Guide for Sterile Compounding Facilities CAG-003-2006 (Revised May 2015). www.cetainternational.org/ceta-application-guides-for-nonmembers. Accessed 25 September 2016.
18. United States Pharmacopeial Convention. General chapter <797> pharmaceutical compounding—sterile preparations. *USP 40–NF 35*; 2017.
19. Critical Point Pearls of Knowledge archive. https://www.criticalpoint.info/tools-resources/sterilecompounding-pearls/. Accessed 25 September 2016.
20. JCR Hazardous Drug Toolkit. www.hazmedsafety.com. Accessed 12 March 2017.
21. United States Pharmacopeial Convention. General chapter <795> pharmaceutical compounding—nonsterile preparations. *USP 40–NF 35*; 2017.
22. United States Pharmacopeial Convention. Proposed revisions to general chapter <797> pharmaceutical compounding—sterile preparations. http://www.usp.org/sites/default/files/usp_pdf/EN/USPNF/usp-gc-797-proposed-revisions-sep-2015.pdf. Accessed 12 March 2017.

APPENDIX – Compounding Hazardous Drugs

LEARNING OBJECTIVES

- Recognize hazardous drugs.
- Discuss the precautions required when working with hazardous drugs.
- Describe the key elements for decontaminating and cleaning areas used for compounding hazardous drugs.
- Discuss the components of a recommended medical surveillance program for those who compound hazardous drugs.

Note: This chapter includes the provisions required by USP Chapter <800> Hazardous Drugs—Handling in Healthcare Settings, which will become official on July 1, 2018. ASHP is updating the *Guidelines on Handling Hazardous Drugs*, which are expected to be published by summer 2017. Recommendations in the revised ASHP guidelines will supersede the requirements in the current recommendations.

Overview

Compounding hazardous drugs requires skill in preparation, as well as protection of the compounding personnel. Injectable oncology agents comprise the majority of hazardous drugs compounded, but agents for other routes of administration and other conditions are also prepared. Competence for compounding hazardous drugs includes written and verbal instruction and review of practices for both sterile and nonsterile compounding. An overview of nonsterile compounding can be found in Chapter 48: Compounding Nonsterile Preparations and an overview of sterile compounding can be found in Chapter 46: Compounding Sterile Preparations (Murdaugh LB, *Competence Assessment Tools for Health-System Pharmacies*, 5th ed., ASHP, 2015).

In addition to the ASHP videos and publications listed in Chapter 46, the video and workbook *Compounding Hazardous Drugs* provides a bridge between didactic instruction and practical skills.[1] Three other resources are critical to knowledge concerning hazardous drugs:

- Guidelines on Handling Hazardous Drugs[2] (www.ashp.org/DocLibrary/BestPractices/PrepGdlHazDrugs.aspx)
- NIOSH Alert: Preventing Occupational Exposure to Antineoplastic and Other Hazardous Drugs in Health Care Settings[3] (www.cdc.gov/niosh/docs/2004-165/pdfs/2004-165.pdf)
- NIOSH List of Antineoplastic and Other Hazardous Drugs in Healthcare Settings, 2016[4] (www.cdc.gov/niosh/topics/antineoplastic/pdf/hazardous-drugs-list_2016-161.pdf)

Completion of written materials is not sufficient to demonstrate competence to compound hazardous drugs. Manipulation of safe and accurate preparations must be demonstrated to a skilled compounder. Competence must be reassessed on a regular basis.

Individuals who compound hazardous drugs must be mentally and physically able to perform accurate calculations and precise and repetitive manipulations; maintain aseptic technique for those preparations intended to be sterile; gown and glove appropriately; clean and decontaminate the compounding areas; and recognize breaks in processes that could result in a hazardous drug preparation, which does not meet quality standards or result in unacceptable risks to patients or personnel.

Definition of a Hazardous Drug

A *hazardous drug* is any drug identified by at least one of the following six characteristics:

1. Carcinogenicity
2. Teratogenicity or developmental toxicity
3. Reproductive toxicity in humans
4. Organ toxicity at low doses in humans or animals
5. Genotoxicity
6. New drugs that mimic existing hazardous drugs in structure or toxicity

Note that the hazardous drugs discussed in this chapter meet the above definition and are hazardous to personnel. However, they are in a different designation than the Environmental Protection Agency (EPA) hazardous materials, which are a hazard to the environment. (See Chapter 18: Hazardous Materials in Murdaugh LB, *Competence Assessment Tools for Health-System Pharmacies*, 5th ed., ASHP, 2015.) There is some overlap between the lists, but the reg-

---

Source: Updated and reprinted with permission from Kienle, PK. Compounding hazardous drugs. In: Murdaugh LB. *Competence Assessment Tools for Health-System Pharmacies*, 5th ed. Bethesda, MD: ASHP; 2015.

ulations stem from different organizations and are directed at different issues.

Each organization must establish its own list of hazardous drugs based on the NIOSH list.[4] The list should be reviewed and revised as formulary changes are made or as nonformulary agents are used for patients, and documentation of the updated list must be done at least annually.

Precautions

When hazardous drugs are manipulated, compounding personnel must be protected from exposure in addition to the requirements for safe and effective preparations for the patient.

The Occupational Safety and Health Administration (OSHA) Hazard Communication Standard requires employers to transmit information concerning workplace hazards to employees.[5] Information must include a safety program, proper labeling, use of safety data sheets (SDS, which were formerly known as material safety data sheets [MSDS]), and employee training.

USP Chapter <797> Pharmaceutical Compounding—Sterile Preparations[6] and USP Chapter <800>[7] provide requirements and recommendations for patient and personnel protection.

Precautions with hazardous drugs are not limited to compounding personnel. Employees who receive, transport, administer, or dispose of the agents must also be aware of the necessary precautions. Inhalation or skin contact and absorption is the most likely way for personnel to be exposed to hazardous drugs. Because manufacturer's vials can be contaminated with trace amounts of hazardous substances, those personnel who receive supplies must follow precautions. All suppliers should provide hazardous drugs in marked and wrapped containers. Personnel who receive and transport hazardous drugs should wear chemotherapy gloves meeting American Society for Testing and Materials (ASTM) standard D6978 when unpacking and transporting hazardous drugs and when wiping supplies and equipment removed from shipping cartons prior to placement in storage bins.

Facility Design

Facilities for Storing and Compounding Hazardous Drugs

The hazardous drug storage or compounding area must have four characteristics[3,7]:

1. It must be a room with fixed walls that is separate from nonhazardous drug storage and preparation.
2. It must be a negative pressure room, which would contain any breakage or spill. USP Chapter <800> requires the pressure to be between 0.01–0.03" wc negative to adjacent areas.
3. It must be vented to the outside of the building.
4. It must have sufficient general exhaust ventilation to dilute potential particles and vapors. Rooms for storage of hazardous drugs, for compounding nonsterile hazardous drugs, or a containment segregated compounding area must have at least 12 air changes per hour (ACPH). Anterooms and buffer rooms for compounding sterile hazardous drugs must have at least 30 ACPH.

Many organizations build their negative pressure sterile buffer area, which requires 30 ACPH, with enough space to also use the area for storage of hazardous drugs. If this is done, care must be taken to ensure that only smooth, impervious containers and shelving (such as cleanable plastic and stainless steel) are used for the storage and that no corrugated cardboard or outer shipping containers are brought into the ante or buffer area. If storage of products is kept in the ante or buffer area, the area must be able to meet the International Organization for Standardization (ISO) 7 air quality standards required of an area for sterile compounding.

Other Attributes of Facilities for Compounding Hazardous Drugs

OSHA recommends an eye wash station in areas where hazardous drugs are manipulated.[8] The American National Standards Institute provides details for the device and its maintenance.[9]

General issues include the following:

- Availability in close proximity to compounding areas used for hazardous drugs
- Plumbed eyewash units connected to cool (not hot) water
- Weekly activation of the station to verify proper operation

Requirements for Compounding Nonsterile Hazardous Drugs

Manipulation of hazardous drugs for oral or other nonsterile routes must be performed in an area separate from the general compounding area. Use of a containment ventilated enclosure such as a Class I biological safety cabinet (BSC) or a ventilated safety enclosure (often informally referred to as a *powder hood*) is recommended. The cabinet or enclosure should be vented to the outside to prevent the hazardous drug particles or vapors from contaminating the area. If it is not externally vented, it must have redundant high-efficiency particulate air (HEPA) filters in series.

Figure 1 provides recommendations for compounding and handling noninjectable hazardous drug dosage forms.

Requirements for Compounding Sterile Hazardous Drugs

See Chapter 46: Compounding Sterile Preparations (Murdaugh LB, *Competence Assessment Tools for Health-System Pharmacies*, 5th ed., ASHP, 2015) for a discussion of components of a sterile compounding area. Hazardous drugs that are intended to be sterile must comply with USP Chapter <797> and USP Chapter <800>.

USP Chapter <800> describes the requirements for preparation areas, which must contain a primary engineering control (PEC), often informally called the *chemo hood*, a secondary engineering control (often called the *IV room*) that is either an IV compounding suite (containing a positive pressure anteroom that serves as a transition area between the general pharmacy area and the site where the hazardous drugs are compounded and a negative pressure buffer room in which the PEC is placed) or a containment segregated compounding area (a negative pressure room in which the PEC is placed).

PECs for compounding hazardous drugs can be a traditional BSC, a compounding aseptic containment isolator (CACI), or a robotic device designed for the preparation of hazardous drugs that meets the definition of a BSC or CACI. PECs used for the preparation of hazardous drugs must not be placed in a positive pressure buffer area used for preparation of nonhazardous drugs.

The National Institute for Occupational Safety and Health (NIOSH) defines a closed system transfer device (CSTD) as one that mechanically prohibits the transfer of environmental contaminants into the system and the escape of hazardous drug or vapor concentrations outside the system. USP Chapter <800> requires use of a CSTD for administration of antineoplastic hazardous drugs when the dosage form allows. Many organizations use a CSTD for preparation of all hazardous drugs. See **Figure 2** for information on use of a Class II BSC and **Figure 3** for information on use of Class III BSCs and CACIs.[2]

Aseptic Technique

Facilities alone cannot prevent exposure to personnel or the environment. Rather, it is dependent on use of proper technique by compounding personnel. *Aseptic technique* refers to a set of specific practices and procedures performed under carefully controlled conditions with the goal of minimizing contamination by pathogens (microbial or fungal contamination). When preparing compounded sterile preparations (CSPs), the compounder must be aware of proper procedures including workflow in the compounding area, placement of products and devices in the PEC, and infection prevention practices including hand hygiene and proper garbing procedures.

Different techniques are used with BSCs, CACIs, and robotic devices. Compounding personnel must have sufficient didactic and practical instruction in the devices and procedures used to be competent to prepare CSPs.

Personal Protective Equipment

Protective clothing, known as *garb*, helps contain the particles and microorganisms produced by compounding personnel. Personal protective equipment (PPE) includes gowns, masks, gloves, hair covers, eye protection, respiratory protection, and shoe covers. **Figure 4** provides recommendations for the use of gloves when handling hazardous drugs.

Key points include the following:

- Use powder-free gloves that meet the ASTM standard D6978 for chemotherapy gloves.
- Follow USP Chapter <797> requirement for use of sterile gloves for the preparation of CSPs.
- Wear two pairs of ASTM-tested chemotherapy gloves for all handling (including receiving, shipping, transporting, compounding, and administration) of hazardous drugs.
- Change gloves every 30 minutes or as recommended by the manufacturer during compounding or immediately if damaged or contaminated.

When using a CACI, place a sterile glove on the outside of the fixed glove assembly. Follow the manufacturer's recommendations for inspecting and changing the fixed glove assembly and gauntlets. The outer ASTM-tested chemotherapy glove (the glove that touches the CSP) must be sterile. The inner glove needs to be an ASTM-tested chemotherapy glove and should be sterile.

Figure 5 provides recommendations for the use of gowns when handling hazardous drugs.[2] Key points include the following:

- Use coated chemotherapy gowns to protect against contamination.
- Change gowns every 3 hours or as recommended by the manufacturer during compounding and immediately when damaged or contaminated.

Two pairs of shoe covers must be donned prior to entering the negative pressure buffer room. Remove the outer pair when leaving the negative pressure buffer room to avoid tracking potential hazardous drug contamination into adjacent areas.

Eye Protection and Respirators

Eye protection is required when working with hazardous drugs. Proper use of BSCs and CACIs provides eye and respiratory protection. Respirators must be worn when handling spills, decontaminating a PEC, and as required by hospital policy. N-95 respirators are effective protection against particles but not gases.

Work Practices

Compounding Procedures

Procedures for CSPs can be found in Chapter 46: Compounding Sterile Preparations (Murdaugh LB, *Competence Assessment Tools for Health-System Pharmacies*, 5th ed., ASHP, 2015). **Figure 6** provides recommendations for working in PECs designed for hazardous drugs.[2] Figure 1 provides recommendations for compounding and handling noninjectable hazardous drug dosage forms.[2]

Decontaminating, Deactivating Substances, and Cleaning the Work Area

In addition to cleaning and disinfecting required for all compounding, working with hazardous drugs also requires deactivation and decontamination of the agents used. There is no single process recommended to deactivate all hazardous drugs. The SDS for each drug used should be reviewed to determine the appropriate agent to use to deactivate and decontaminate an area used for compounding hazardous drugs. Many SDSs recommend decontamination with sodium hypochlorite (bleach). Other commercial products are also available, including those designed for decontaminating hazardous drugs. Alcohol does not deactivate hazardous drugs and can spread contamination if used prior to deactivation.

BSCs and CACIs should be cleaned as detailed in the manufacturers' recommendations. Full garb must be worn while performing this process. Decontaminating, deactivating, cleaning, and disinfecting include the following steps:

- Decontaminate the PEC and deactivate the hazardous drug using an agent recommended in the SDS (such as 2% sodium hypochlorite or other EPA-approved oxidizer intended for use with hazardous drugs). If sodium hypochlorite is used, deactivate the sodium hypochlorite (and some hazardous drugs) with 1% sodium thiosulfate, rinse with sufficient amount of sterile water, or immediately follow with the next step to remove the sodium hypochlorite.
- Clean the area with a germicidal detergent.
- Disinfect the area with sterile 70% isopropyl alcohol.

The decontamination process should be used prior to starting the day's operation, at regular intervals during compounding, in the case of a spill or suspected contamination, and when the shift's work is completed.

Spills

All personnel who receive, transport, compound, or administer hazardous drugs must be trained in actions to take in case of a spill or breakage. **Figure 7** lists the recommended contents of a spill kit.[2] The kit must be available in all areas where hazardous drugs are received, stored, compounded, or administered. **Figure 8** lists recommendations for spill cleanup procedures.[2] Your organization should have a detailed procedure, including specific departments to contact if a spill or breakage occurs.

Direct Skin or Eye Contact

Figure 9 provides recommendations for immediate treatment of personnel with direct skin or eye contact with hazardous drugs, including flushing the affected eye with water or isotonic eyewash in a continuous stream for at least 15 minutes.[2]

Disposal

The federal Resource Conservation and Recovery Act (RCRA) was enacted in 1976 to provide a means for tracking hazardous waste. RCRA defines hazardous waste as substances that are considered detrimental to the environment and must be segregated for special waste management. RCRA states hazardous waste cannot be discarded into waste water systems (e.g., sewers, drains) or landfills. Some hazardous drugs are defined as hazardous waste under this act. Follow your health-system's policy concerning disposal and segregation of all hazardous drugs.

Medical Surveillance Program

NIOSH has defined a medical surveillance program for healthcare workers who are exposed to hazardous drugs.[10] Healthcare organizations are expected to have in place a comprehensive approach to worker safety and health, including the following:

- Engineering controls
- Good work practices
- Availability of PPE
- Follow-up for workers who had health changes or had a significant exposure

Elements of the medical surveillance program include the following, performed at hire and periodically:

- Reproductive and general health questionnaire
- Laboratory studies, including complete blood counts, urinalysis, and other appropriate tests
- Physical examination

References

1. Power LA, Jorgenson J. *Safe Handling of Hazardous Drugs Video Training Program*. Bethesda, MD: American Society of Health-System Pharmacists; 2006.
2. American Society of Health-System Pharmacists (ASHP). ASHP guidelines on handling hazardous drugs. *Am J Health-Syst Pharm*. 2006; 63(Jun 15):1172-1193.
3. National Institute for Occupational Safety and Health (NIOSH). NIOSH alert: preventing occupational exposure to antineoplastic and other hazardous drugs in healthcare settings. NIOSH publication number 2004-165. September 2004. www.cdc.gov/niosh/docs/2004-165. Accessed March 2, 2017.
4. National Institute for Occupational Safety and Health (NIOSH). NIOSH list of antineoplastic and other hazardous drugs in healthcare settings 2016. NIOSH publication number 2016-161. September 2016. www.cdc.gov/niosh/docs/2016-161/. Accessed March 2, 2017.
5. Occupational Safety and Health Administration (OSHA). Hazard communication standard. www.osha.gov/pls/oshaweb/owadisp.show_document?p_table=STANDARDS&p_id=10099. Accessed March 2, 2017.
6. The U.S. Pharmacopeial Convention (USP). Chapter <797>. Pharmaceutical compounding—sterile preparations. In: *United States Pharmacopeia*, 40th rev./*National Formulary*, 35th ed. Rockville, MD: USP; 2017.
7. The U.S. Pharmacopeial Convention (USP). Chapter <800>. Hazardous drugs—handling in healthcare settings. In: *United States Pharmacopeia*, 40th rev./*National Formulary*, 35th ed. Rockville, MD: USP; 2017.
8. Occupational Safety and Health Administration (OSHA). Controlling occupational exposure to hazardous drugs. www.osha.gov/SLTC/hazardousdrugs/controlling_occex_hazardousdrugs.html. Accessed March 2, 2017.
9. American National Standards Institute (ANSI). Emergency eyewash and shower equipment, ANSI Z358.1-2014. www.ansi.org. Accessed March 2, 2017.
10. National Institute for Occupational Safety and Health (NIOSH). Medical surveillance for health care workers exposed to hazardous drugs, NIOSH publication number 2013-103. November 2012. www.cdc.gov/niosh/docs/wp-solutions/2013-103/. Accessed March 2, 2017.

Resources

- ASHP. ASHP guidelines on compounding sterile preparations. *Am J Health-Syst Pharm*. 2014; 71(2):145-166. www.ashp.org/DocLibrary/BestPractices/PrepGdlCSP.aspx. Accessed March 2, 2017.
- ASHP. ASHP Sterile Compounding Resources Center. www.ashp.org/menu/PracticePolicy/ResourceCenters/Compounding. Accessed March 2, 2017.
- Conner TH, McDiarmid MA. Preventing occupational exposures to antineoplastic drugs in health care settings. *CA Cancer J Clin*. 2006; 56(6):354-365.
- Davis KM, Benner KW. Potential complications of exposure to cytotoxic agents for caregivers. *Am J Health-Syst Pharm*. 2003; 38:1097-1102.
- Goldspiel B, Hoffman JM, Friffith NL, et al.; American Society of Health-System Pharmacists (ASHP). ASHP guidelines on preventing medication errors with chemotherapy and biotherapy. *Am J Health-Syst Pharm*. 2015;72c6-35. www.ashp.org/DocLibrary/BestPractices/MedMisGdlAntineo.aspx. Accessed March 2, 2017.
- Power LA. Hazardous drugs as compounded sterile preparations. In: Buchanan EC, Schneider PJ, eds. *Compounding Sterile Preparations*. 3rd ed. Bethesda, MD: ASHP; 2009:79-97.

Competence Checklist

Name: _____ Date: _____

Knowledge and Skills	Yes	No
Recognizes that cytotoxic and other hazardous medications must not be prepared in a PEC designed for use with nonhazardous drugs. *Note:* The organization may entity-exempt some dosage forms of nonantineoplastic and reproductive-only hazards from this requirement.		
Demonstrates knowledge of preparation of nonsterile hazardous medications including packaging activities		
Recognizes that hazardous medications must be prepared only in a BSC or CACI or robotic device designed for compounding sterile hazardous drugs		
Recognizes that the BSC or CACI is dedicated only to preparing hazardous medications		
Recognizes that if the exhaust fan on a BSC or CACI is turned off, the cabinet must be decontaminated, cleaned, and disinfected before reuse		
Recognizes that a BSC or CACI must be serviced and certified by a qualified technician every 6 months and when it is moved, repaired, or if the HEPA filter is contaminated by a spill		
Demonstrates proper infection control (removes jewelry, ties long hair back, washes hands with approved cleaning agents, etc.)		
States the organization's requirements for PPE.		
Wears appropriate protective equipment properly (e.g., ASTM-tested chemotherapy gloves, impervious gown, mask, hair and shoe covers)		
Cleans and disinfects the BSC or CACI at the beginning of the work shift, as appropriate during compounding, and at the end of each shift		
Decontaminates, deactivates, cleans, and disinfects the BSC or CACI with appropriate agents and in the proper order, working from the top to the bottom or as according to manufacturer's recommendations		
Correctly performs all required calculations prior to compounding preparation		
Uses appropriate safeguards that may reduce the potential for medication errors involving chemotherapy agents (e.g., independent double checks)		
Collects correct medications, solutions, and supplies; inspects all components, including vials, ampules, IV bags for damage/contamination and expiration date before compounding		
Places appropriate medications and supplies in the BSC or CACI prior to compounding; demonstrates proper placement of items to prevent blocking air flow; keeps nonessential items outside PEC		
Checks labels both prior to and after compounding to ensure medications and solutions being used agree		
Maintains BSC glass safety shield at appropriate opening height (based on manufacturer recommendations and confirmation by certifier) during admixture operations		

Demonstrates understanding of air flow in C-PEC, maintains flow of clean air over objects in C-PEC, does not interrupt air flow; places only hands and arms in BSC		
Does not utilize outer area of BSC opening (based on manufacturer's recommendations and confirmation by certifier), work too close to sides of C-PEC, or block air intake grills during admixture preparation		
Does not take hands out of C-PEC or leave the C-PEC during admixture preparation		
Does not compromise air flow in the ante or buffer area		
Does not touch or contaminate any component that must remain sterile during aseptic admixture preparation		
Reviews Master Formulation Record prior to mixing		
Performs all work on plastic-backed paper mat placed on the work surface		
Demonstrates proper swabbing and entering of vials, ampules, and bags		
Correctly uses appropriate transfer devices (CSTDs, Luer-Lok syringes, filter needles, vented needles, dispensing pins, etc.)		
Reconstitutes powders using proper technique		
Uses negative pressure technique during reconstitution and withdrawal of medication; does not aspirate at any time		
After preparation, inspects solution for cores, precipitates, particulate matter, etc.		
Wipes admixture container with approved decontamination agent before labeling the container		
Removes outer gloves, then affixes appropriate labels to admixture container including auxiliary and chemotherapy hazard labels; places container in a sealable plastic bag prior to removal from the PEC		
Disposes of all used equipment and waste in appropriate hazardous waste disposal containers; seals and wipes waste containers prior to removal from the PEC		
After completion of operations in the PEC, removes PPE (e.g., hair cover, gown, shoe covers, gloves) and places in appropriate waste container; performs hand hygiene after completion of compounding activities		
Documents preparation in appropriate records (e.g., patients' medication profiles, compounding records)		
Demonstrates knowledge of proper procedure for reporting and cleaning up hazardous medication spills both within and outside the PEC; correctly verbalizes location of materials used to clean up spills (e.g., spill kit)		
NOTES		

Competence certified by:_____ Date:_____

Competency Assessment Exam

Name: _____ Date: _____

___ 1. When reconstituting and withdrawing chemotherapy medications from vials, aerosol droplets may be generated. This can be minimized or eliminated by using _____.
   a. Negative pressure technique
   b. Luer-Lok syringes
   c. Closed-system transfer devices (CSTDs)
   d. a and c

___ 2. All of the following statements is true *except* _____.
   a. Personnel preparing hazardous medications should wear protective apparel.
   b. Personnel should wash hands after preparing chemotherapy medications.
   c. Syringes or admixtures containing chemotherapy agents should have distinctive chemotherapy cautionary labeling.
   d. Gowns and gloves worn in preparing chemotherapy medications can be used for several days.

___ 3. Gloves used in the preparation of chemotherapy must be _____.
   a. Disposable
   b. Powdered to facilitate removal
   c. Specified as ASTM-tested chemotherapy gloves
   d. a and c

___ 4. Gowns and gloves worn while working in the chemotherapy preparation area can be worn while working in other medication preparation areas.
   a. True
   b. False

___ 5. When wearing double gloves, _____.
   a. The gown cuffs should be tucked over both gloves
   b. The gown cuffs should be tucked under both gloves
   c. The inner glove should be worn under the gown cuff and the outer glove should be worn over the gown cuff
   d. It makes no difference if gown cuffs are worn over or under the gloves

___ 6. Hazardous medication warning labels are required on _____.
   a. Shelves and bins where hazardous medications are stored
   b. Syringes, vials, IV bottles, and IV bags containing chemotherapy preparations
   c. Waste containers for disposal of hazardous drugs
   d. All of the above

___ 7. When reconstituting a hazardous powder, the needle should be removed and the vial shaken before withdrawing the liquid.
   a. True
   b. False

___ 8. After preparing a chemotherapy medication, the product should be wiped and placed in a sealable plastic bag before removal from the BSC.

    a. True
    b. False

___ 9. Excess amounts of hazardous medications drawn into a syringe should be _____.
    a. Squirted down the sink drain
    b. Squirted into the chemotherapy waste container
    c. Injected back into the vial before removing the needle
    d. Any of the above techniques are acceptable

___ 10. Which of the following types of PECs can be used for preparing sterile hazardous medications?
    a. Ventilated safety enclosure
    b. Biological safety cabinet (BSC)
    c. Horizontal laminar air flow workbench
    d. Compounding aseptic isolator (CAI)

___ 11. When decontaminating a BSC, _____.
    a. Protective apparel must be worn
    b. Media fill testing should be performed
    c. Rinse water can be poured down the sink
    d. a and c

___ 12. BSCs and CACIs must be serviced and certified _____.
    a. Every month
    b. Every 6 months
    c. Every year
    d. Prior to accreditation surveys

___ 13. If a BSC is turned off, it must be decontaminated before reuse.
    a. True
    b. False

___ 14. BSCs must be decontaminated _____.
    a. Regularly as specified by facility policy
    b. When the cabinet is moved or serviced
    c. When a spill occurs
    d. All of the above

___ 15. A BSC is cleaned from the top to bottom.
    a. True
    b. False

___ 16. When preparing hazardous medications in a BSC, the glass shield must be raised _____.
    a. All the way
    b. As recommended by the manufacturer and confirmed by the certifier
    c. No more than 6 inches
    d. Depending on the height of the operator

___ 17. Spill kits _____.
    a. Should be available only from the facility's central supply room
    b. Should be kept wherever chemotherapy agents are handled
    c. Contain supplies needed to clean a hazardous drug spill
    d. b and c

___ 18. During hazardous drug compounding, gloves should be _____.
   a. Used for one shift
   b. Changed every batch
   c. Changed every 30 minutes or as recommended by the manufacturer
   d. Changed every 3 hours or as recommended by the manufacturer

___ 19. During hazardous drug compounding, gowns should be _____.
   a. Used for one shift
   b. Changed every batch
   c. Changed every 30 minutes or as recommended by the manufacturer
   d. Changed every 3 hours or as recommended by the manufacturer

___ 20. Cleaning hazardous drug preparation areas requires decontamination and deactivation prior to cleaning and disinfecting.
   a. True
   b. False

_____   _____
Competence certified by   Date

Answer Key

1. d. CSTDs provide a supplemental engineering control to reduce risk of contamination. Negative pressure technique must be used if CSTDs are not used.
2. d. Work practices including hand hygiene and appropriate PPE must be followed. Distinctive cautionary labeling should be used. Garb used when mixing chemotherapy must be discarded when leaving the hazardous drug compounding area.
3. d. Disposable chemotherapy gloves that meet ASTM standard D6978 are required. Powdered gloves are not permitted.
4. False. PPE used when mixing chemotherapy must be removed and discarded when leaving the hazardous drug compounding area.
5. c. Placing the inner glove under the gown cuff and the outer glove over the gown cuff provides the best protection, and this allows removal of the outer glove without compromising the protection provided by the gown and inner glove.
6. d. All areas where hazardous medications are stored or disposed require warning labels.
7. False. Technique that minimizes the potential for droplets of hazardous medications to escape from a closed container must be used.
8. True. Hazardous drug preparations must be contained in a sealable plastic bag prior to removal from the PEC to minimize the possibility of contamination outside the BSC or CACI.
9. c. Unused hazardous drugs must be contained, such as in the vial. Never expel unused hazardous drugs down a drain or into an open waste container.
10. b. Sterile hazardous drugs can be compounded only in either a BSC or a CACI.
11. a. PPE must be worn when decontaminating a BSC.
12. b. All PECs must be certified every 6 months.
13. True. BSCs and CACIs should be powered on continuously. If the power has been off, the PEC must be decontaminated, cleaned, and disinfected prior to use.
14. d. The PEC must be decontaminated whenever there is a risk that it might have been contaminated. This would include anytime a spill occurs or if the cabinet was moved. Additionally, the facility policy requirements must be followed.
15. True. The BSC or CACI should be cleaned from top to bottom and from back to front.
16. b. The manufacturer's information and the results of the certification of the particular BSC will determine the height of the glass shield.
17. d. Spill kits must be available wherever hazardous drugs are located and must include all the equipment that would be required to clean a spill.
18. c. Outer gloves should be changed every 30 minutes or as recommended by manufacturer or when contaminated or suspected of being contaminated.
19. d. Gowns should be changed following manufacturer's recommendations or every 3 hours if no manufacturer's information is available.
20. True. Cleaning hazardous drug preparation areas requires decontamination and deactivation prior to cleaning and disinfecting.

FIGURE 1. *Recommendations for Compounding and Handling Noninjectable Hazardous Drug Dosage Forms*

- Hazardous drugs should be labeled or otherwise identified as such to prevent improper handling.
- Tablet and capsule forms of hazardous drugs should not be placed in automated counting machines, which subject them to stress and may introduce powdered contaminants into the work area.
- During routine handling of noninjectable hazardous drugs and contaminated equipment, workers should wear two pairs of gloves that meet the ASTM standard for chemotherapy gloves.
- Counting and pouring of hazardous drugs should be done carefully, and clean equipment should be dedicated for use with these drugs.
- Contaminated equipment should be cleaned initially with wipes saturated with sterile water; decontaminated, then further cleaned with detergent, sodium hypochlorite solution, and neutralizer; and then rinsed. The wipes and rinse should be contained and disposed of as contaminated waste.
- Crushing tablets or opening capsules should be avoided when possible; liquid formulations should be used whenever possible.
- During the compounding of hazardous drugs (e.g., crushing, dissolving, or preparing a solution or an ointment), workers should wear nonpermeable gowns and double chemotherapy gloves. Compounding must take place in a ventilated cabinet.
- Compounding nonsterile forms of hazardous drugs in equipment designated for sterile products must be undertaken with care. Appropriate containment, deactivation, cleaning, and disinfection techniques must be utilized.
- Hazardous drugs should be dispensed in the final dose and form whenever possible. Most unit-of-use containers exhibit some spillage during preparation or use. Caution must be exercised when using these devices.
- Bulk containers of liquid hazardous drugs, as well as specially packaged commercial hazardous drugs (e.g., Neoral [manufactured by Novartis]), must be handled carefully to avoid spills. These containers should be dispensed and maintained in sealable plastic bags to contain any inadvertent contamination.
- Disposal of unused or unusable noninjectable dosage forms of hazardous drugs should be performed in the same manner as for hazardous injectable dosage forms and waste.

ASTM = American Society for Testing and Materials.

Source: Adapted from and originally published in American Society of Health-System Pharmacists (ASHP). ASHP guidelines on handling hazardous drugs. *Am J Health-Syst Pharm.* 2006; 63(Jun 15):1172-1193. © 2006, American Society of Health-System Pharmacists, Inc. All rights reserved.

FIGURE 2. *Recommendations for Use of Class II Biological Safety Cabinets (BSCs)*

- The use of a Class II BSC must be accompanied by a stringent program of work practices, including training, demonstrated competence, contamination reduction, and decontamination.
- Only a Class II BSC with outside exhaust should be used for compounding hazardous drugs. Total exhaust is required if the hazardous drug is known to be volatile.
- Consider using closed system transfer devices while compounding hazardous drugs in a Class II BSC; evidence documents a decrease in drug contaminants inside a Class II BSC when such devices are used.
- Reduce the hazardous drug contamination burden in the Class II BSC by wiping down hazardous drug vials before placing them in the BSC.

Source: Adapted from and originally published in American Society of Health-System Pharmacists (ASHP). ASHP guidelines on handling hazardous drugs. *Am J Health-Syst Pharm.* 2006; 63(Jun 15):1172-1193. © 2006, American Society of Health-System Pharmacists, Inc. All rights reserved.

FIGURE 3. *Recommendations for Use of Class III BSCs and Compounding Isolators*

- Only a ventilated cabinet designed to protect workers and adjacent personnel from exposure and to provide an aseptic environment may be used to compound sterile hazardous drugs.
- Only ventilated cabinets that are designed to contain aerosolized drug product within the cabinet should be used to compound hazardous drugs.
- The use of a Class III BSC or compounding isolator must be accompanied by a stringent program of work practices, including operator training and demonstrated competence, contamination reduction, and decontamination.
- Decontamination of the Class III BSC or compounding isolator must be done in a way that contains any hazardous drug surface contamination during the cleaning process.
- Appropriate decontamination within the cabinet must be completed before the cabinet is accessed via pass-throughs or removable front panels.
- Gloves or gauntlets must not be replaced before completion of appropriate decontamination within the cabinet.
- Surface decontamination of final preparations must be done before labeling and placing into the pass-through.
- Final preparations must be placed into a transport bag while in the pass-through for removal from the cabinet.

BSC = biological safety cabinet.

Source: Adapted from and originally published in American Society of Health-System Pharmacists (ASHP). ASHP guidelines on handling hazardous drugs. *Am J Health-Syst Pharm.* 2006; 63(Jun 15):1172-1193. © 2006, American Society of Health-System Pharmacists, Inc. All rights reserved.

FIGURE 4. *Recommendations for Use of Gloves*

- Wear chemotherapy gloves for all activities involving hazardous drugs. Gloves must be worn during any handling of hazardous drug shipping cartons or drug vials, compounding and administration of hazardous drugs, handling of hazardous drug waste or waste from patients recently treated with hazardous drugs, and cleanup of hazardous drug spills.
- Select powder-free, high-quality gloves made of latex, nitrile, polyurethane, neoprene, or other materials that meet the ASTM standard for chemotherapy gloves (D6978).
- Inspect gloves for visible defects.
- Disinfect gloves with sterile 70% alcohol or other appropriate disinfectant before performing any aseptic compounding activity.
- Change gloves every 30 minutes during compounding or as recommended by the manufacturer, and immediately when damaged or contaminated.
- Remove outer gloves after wiping down final preparation but before labeling or removing the preparation from the BSC.
- Outer gloves must be placed in a containment bag while in the C-PEC.
- In a compounding isolator, a sterile glove must be worn over the fixed-glove assembly.
- In a compounding isolator, fixed gloves or gauntlets must be surface cleaned after compounding is completed to avoid spreading hazardous drug contamination to other surfaces.
- Clean gloves (e.g., the clean inner gloves worn by compounding personnel) should be used to surface decontaminate the final preparation, place the label onto the final preparation, and place it into the pass-through.
- Don fresh gloves to complete the final check, place preparation into a clean transport bag, and remove the bag from the pass-through.
- Wash hands before donning and after removing gloves.
- Remove gloves with care to avoid contamination. Specific procedures for removal must be established and followed.
- Change gloves after administering a dose of hazardous drugs or when leaving the immediate administration area.
- Dispose of contaminated gloves as contaminated waste.

ASTM = American Society for Testing and Materials; C-PEC = containment primary engineering control.

Source: Adapted from and originally published in American Society of Health-System Pharmacists (ASHP). ASHP guidelines on handling hazardous drugs. *Am J Health-Syst Pharm.* 2006; 63(Jun 15):1172-1193. © 2006, American Society of Health-System Pharmacists, Inc. All rights reserved.

FIGURE 5. *Recommendations for Use of Gowns*

- Gowns should be worn during compounding, during administration, when handling waste from patients recently treated with hazardous drugs, and when cleaning up spills of hazardous drugs.
- Select disposable gowns of material tested to be protective against the hazardous drugs to be used.
- Coated gowns must be worn no longer than 3 hours or as required by the manufacturer during compounding and changed immediately when damaged or contaminated.
- Remove gowns with care to avoid spreading contamination. Specific procedures for removal must be established and followed.
- Dispose of gowns immediately upon removal.
- Contain and dispose of contaminated gowns as contaminated waste.
- Wash hands after removing and disposing of gowns.

Source: Adapted from and originally published in American Society of Health-System Pharmacists (ASHP). ASHP guidelines on handling hazardous drugs. *Am J Health-Syst Pharm.* 2006; 63(Jun 15):1172-1193. © 2006, American Society of Health-System Pharmacists, Inc. All rights reserved.

FIGURE 6. *Recommendations for Working in BSCs and Compounding Isolators*

- The use of a C-PEC or isolator must be accompanied by a stringent program of work practices, including operator training and demonstrated competence, contamination reduction, and decontamination.
- Do not place unnecessary items in the work area of the cabinet or compounding isolator where hazardous drug contamination from compounding may settle on them.
- Do not overcrowd the BSC or CACI.
- Gather all needed supplies before beginning compounding. Avoid exiting and reentering the work area of the BSC or compounding isolator (CACI).
- Appropriate handling of the preparation in the BSC or pass-through of the isolator, including wiping with sterile 70% alcohol, is necessary for aseptic compounding.
- Reduce the hazardous drug contamination burden in the BSC or CACI by wiping down hazardous drug vials before placing them in the BSC or CACI.
- Do not place transport bags in the BSC or the CACI work chamber during compounding to avoid inadvertent contamination of the outside surface of the bag.
- Final preparations should be surface decontaminated within the BSC or CACI and placed into the transport bags in the BSC or in the CACI pass-through, taking care not to contaminate the outside of the transport bag.
- Decontaminate the work surface of the BSC or CACI before and after compounding per the manufacturer's recommendations.
- Decontaminate all surfaces of the BSC or CACI at the end of the batch, day, or shift, as appropriate to the workflow. Typically, a BSC or CACI in use 24 hours a day would require decontamination two or three times daily. Disinfect the BSC or CACI before compounding a dose or batch of sterile hazardous drugs.
- Wipe down the outside of the C-PEC front opening and the floor in front of it with detergent, sodium hypochlorite solution, and neutralizer at least daily.
- Seal and then decontaminate surfaces of waste and sharps containers before removing from the BSC or CACI.
- Decontamination is required after any spill in the BSC or CACI during compounding.
- Seal all contaminated materials (e.g., wipes, towels, wash or rinse water) in bags or plastic containers and discard as contaminated waste.
- Decontamination of the C-PEC must be done in a way that contains any hazardous drug surface contamination during the cleaning process.
- Appropriate decontamination within the C-PEC must be completed before the cabinet is accessed via the pass-throughs or removable front panels.

APPENDIX – Compounding Hazardous Drugs

- Gloves or gauntlets must not be replaced before completion of appropriate decontamination within the CACI.
- Surface decontamination of final preparations must be done before labeling and placing into the pass-through of the CACI.
- Final preparations must be placed into a transport bag while in the pass-through for removal from the cabinet.

BSC = biological safety cabinet; CACI = compounding aseptic containment isolator; C-PEC = containment primary engineering control.

Source: Adapted from and originally published in American Society of Health-System Pharmacists (ASHP). ASHP guidelines on handling hazardous drugs. *Am J Health-Syst Pharm.* 2006; 63(Jun 15):1172-1193. © 2006, American Society of Health-System Pharmacists, Inc. All rights reserved.

FIGURE 7. *Recommended Contents of Hazardous Drug Spill Kit*

- Sufficient supplies to absorb a spill of about 1,000 mL (volume of one IV bag or bottle)
- Appropriate PPE to protect the worker during cleanup, including two pairs of disposable chemotherapy gloves (one outer pair of heavy utility gloves and one pair of inner gloves); nonpermeable, disposable protective garments (coveralls or gown and shoe covers); and face shield
- Absorbent, plastic-backed sheets or spill pads
- Disposable toweling
- At least two sealable, thick plastic hazardous waste disposal bags (prelabeled with an appropriate warning label)
- One disposable scoop for collecting glass fragments
- One puncture-resistant container for glass fragments

IV = intravenous; PPE = personal protective equipment.

Source: Adapted from and originally published in American Society of Health-System Pharmacists (ASHP). ASHP guidelines on handling hazardous drugs. *Am J Health-Syst Pharm.* 2006; 63(Jun 15):1172-1193. © 2006, American Society of Health-System Pharmacists, Inc. All rights reserved.

FIGURE 8. *Recommendations for Spill Cleanup Procedure*

General

- Assess the size and scope of the spill. Call for trained help, if necessary.
- Spills that cannot be contained by two spill kits may require outside assistance.
- Post signs to limit access to spill area.
- Obtain spill kit and respirator.
- Don PPE, including inner and outer gloves and respirator.
- Once fully garbed, contain spill using spill kit.
- Carefully remove any broken glass fragments and place them in a puncture-resistant container.
- Absorb liquids with spill pads.
- Absorb powder with damp disposable pads or soft toweling.
- Spill cleanup should proceed progressively from areas of lesser to greater contamination.
- Completely remove and place all contaminated material in the disposal bags.
- Rinse the area with water and then clean with detergent, sodium hypochlorite solution (or other appropriate decontamination agent), and neutralizer.
- Rinse the area several times and place all materials used for containment and cleanup in disposal bags. Seal bags and place them in the appropriate final container for disposal as hazardous waste.
- Carefully remove all PPE using the inner gloves. Place all disposable PPE into disposal bags. Seal bags and place them into the appropriate final container.

Continued on next page

- Remove inner gloves; contain in a small, sealable bag; and then place into the appropriate final container for disposal as hazardous waste.
- Wash hands thoroughly with soap and water.
- Once a spill has been initially cleaned, have the area recleaned by environmental services.

Spills in a BSC or Compounding Isolator

- Spills occurring in a BSC or isolator should be cleaned up immediately.
- Obtain a spill kit if the volume of the spill exceeds 30 mL or the contents of one drug vial or ampul.
- Utility gloves (from spill kit) should be worn to remove broken glass in a BSC or CACI. Care must be taken not to damage the fixed-glove assembly in the CACI.
- Place glass fragments in the puncture-resistant hazardous drug waste container located in the C-PEC or discard into the appropriate waste receptacle of the isolator.
- Thoroughly clean and decontaminate the C-PEC.
- Clean and decontaminate the drain spillage trough located under the C-PEC.
- If the spill results in liquid being introduced onto the HEPA filter or if powdered aerosol contaminates the "clean side" of the HEPA filter, use of the BSC or CACI should be suspended until the equipment has been decontaminated and the HEPA filter replaced.

BSC = biological safety cabinet; CACI = compounding aseptic containment isolator; C-PEC = containment primary engineering control; HEPA = high-efficiency particulate air; PPE = personal protective equipment.

Source: Adapted from and originally published in American Society of Health-System Pharmacists (ASHP). ASHP guidelines on handling hazardous drugs. *Am J Health-Syst Pharm.* 2006; 63(Jun 15):1172-1193. © 2006, American Society of Health-System Pharmacists, Inc. All rights reserved.

FIGURE 9. *OSHA-Recommended Steps for Immediate Treatment of Workers with Direct Skin or Eye Contact with Hazardous Drugs*

- Call for help, if needed.
- Immediately remove contaminated clothing.
- Flood affected eye with water or isotonic eyewash for at least 15 minutes.
- Clean affected skin with soap and water; rinse thoroughly.
- Obtain medical attention.
- Document exposure in employee's medical record and medical surveillance log.
- Supplies for emergency treatment (e.g., soap, eyewash, sterile saline for irrigation) should be immediately located in any area where hazardous drugs are compounded or administered.

OSHA = Occupational Safety and Health Administration.

Source: Adapted from and originally published in American Society of Health-System Pharmacists (ASHP). ASHP guidelines on handling hazardous drugs. *Am J Health-Syst Pharm.* 2006; 63(Jun 15):1172-1193. © 2006, American Society of Health-System Pharmacists, Inc. All rights reserved.

INDEX

A

Acrylic glove box, 77
Active pharmaceutical ingredients (APIs), 4, 20, 23, 59, 88, 107
    compounding policies for, 107-117
    manipulation of, 90
    storage of, 23, 107
    weighing of, 113
Administration, of hazardous drugs, 9, 131-133
    personal protective equipment for, 39
Administrative controls, 17
Agent additions, 3
Air changes per hour (ACPH), 85, 91
Airborne exposure, 49
Alcohol, 136, 137
    application, 115
    gel, 116
    spray, 115
Alert on Preventing Occupational Exposure to Antineoplastic and Other Hazardous Drugs in Health Care Settings, 3
Alternative containment, 27, 36
Ambulatory patient finished dosage forms to, 128
American Society for Testing and Materials (ASTM)
    D6978, 35, 42-44, 56, 152
    F739, 42, 44
American Society of Heating, Refrigerating, and Air-Conditioning Engineers (ASHRAE), 74, 76, 110
Anterooms, 37-38, 78, 94-95, 96, 99
Antineoplastic agents, 19, 23, 27
    compounding, 64, 88, 97-98
    compounding policies, 107-117
    CSDTs and, 83
    gowns and, 44-45
    injectable, 61
    manipulation of, 90
    storage and compounding, 64
Appendix 1: Acronyms, 9
Appendix 2: Examples of Design for HD Compounding Areas, 10
Appendix 3: Types of Biological Safety Cabinets, 10
Aseptic technique, 153-154
ASHP, 3
    Guidelines on Handling Hazardous Drugs, 18, 107, 146
    Technical Assistance Bulletin on Handling Cytotoxic and Hazardous Drugs, 18
Assessment of Risk, 12, 13, 19, 23-28
    allowances, 24
    approach to, 23-24
    HD inclusions, 24
    reporting, documentation, 27
    review, 27
    spreadsheet, 24, 25-26
Automated counting, packaging machines, 27
Automated dispensing cabinets, 65, 127
Azathioprine, 126

B

Bacillus Calmette-Guérin, 114, 117
Batching chemo pre-meds, 78
Beta-lactam antibiotics, 3
Bevacizumab, 20
Beyond-use date, 77, 79, 90, 95-96, 104, 121
Biological safety cabinet (BSC), 5, 28, 40, 72, 77-81, 124, 164-165
    Class II, 162
    Class III, 163
    classes, 79-80
    double-gloving and, 43, 44
    exhaust, 80, 96
    nonsterile compounding in, 74, 75
    respiratory protection for, 49
    sterile compounding in, 76
Bleach, 136, 137
Breast-feeding employee, 29
Broken containers, 56, 58

Buffer room, 94, 96
    drug storage, refrigerators in, 67
    garb in, 55
Bulk packaging, 5

C

Capsule opening, 124
Carcinogenic drugs, 19
Carmustine, 44
Carousel storage, 65
Cart pass-through, 93, 101-102
Ceiling caulking, 97
Centers for Disease Control and Prevention (CDC), 35
Centers for Medicare & Medicaid Services (CMS)
    Hospital Conditions of Participation, 21
Cetuximab, 20
Chemotherapy administration, shoe covers, 47
Chemotherapy bag, 127
    packaging, 54, 55
Chemotherapy gloves, 28, 35-36, 39-43, 56, 128, 163
    changing, 44
    permeability of, 44
Chemotherapy gowns, 44-45
Chemotherapy hood, 32
    cleaning, 135
Chemotherapy items check, 114
Chemotherapy preparations, 29
Chemotherapy vial storage, 63
Classified room, 89
Cleaning, 135-138, 154
    guidelines, 136
    monitoring, 138
Cleanroom, 79, 89, 96, 146
Cleanroom suite, 71, 77
Clonazepam, 21
Closed system drug-transfer devices (CSTDs), 4, 71, 83-84, 115-116
    compounding in, 84
    nursing and, 132-133
Coated tablets, capsules, 18
Community pharmacies, 11
    NIOSH list and, 74-75
    storage in, 67

Competence
    checklist, 156-157
    documentation, 31-32
Competence Assessment exam, 158-160
    answer key, 161
Competence Assessment Tools for Health-System Pharmacies, 31-32, 133
Compliance, 4, 11
    enforcement, 14
Compounding, 9, 37, 151
    area design, 104-105
    covered, 11
    noninjectables, 162
    powders, 38
    precautions, 152
    procedures, 154
    training, 31-32
Compounding aseptic containment isolator (CACI), 5, 38, 40, 72, 77-81, 97
    CSTDs and, 83
    double-gloving in, 43, 44
    not externally vented, 75
    respiratory protection in, 49
    sterile compounding in, 76, 78
Compounding facilities design, 82-93
    minimum requirements, 85-87
Compounding isolator, 40, 101, 163-165
    ante-chamber, 101
Conjugated monoclonals, 20
Container
    broken, damaged, 56, 58
    identification, 58
    labeling, 54
Containment, 123
    precautions, 28
    strategies, 4-5, 17, 23
Containment primary engineering control (C-PEC), 37, 38, 71, 72
    certification, 93-94
    cleaning, 137
    environmental monitoring, 139-141
    hood, 92
    nonsterile compounding in, 73-76
    sterile compounding in, 76-81
Containment secondary engineering control (C-SEC), 71, 72-73, 93-99
    certification, 93-94

Containment segregated compounding area (C-SCA), 4, 54, 64, 73, 87-90, 96, 98-100
   donning, doffing order from, 41
   perimeter for, 99-100
   sink placement and, 92
Containment ventilated enclosure (CVE), 54, 71, 72, 74, 94, 98
Contaminated products, 18
Contamination, 140-141
Controlled Environment Testing Association (CETA), 74, 95
   Application Guides, 94
Corrugated cardboard, 115
Counting, 28, 124
Counting tray, 126
Cyclophosphamide, 140

D

Damaged containers, 56, 58
Deactivating, Decontaminating, Cleaning, and Disinfecting, 9
Deactivation, 136, 137, 154
Decontamination, 128, 135-138, 154
   agents, 136
Designated person, 30-31, 140, 147
   training, 31
Developmental toxins, 19
Diclofenac gel, 21
Direct skin/eye contact, 154, 166
Disinfecting agents, 136
Disinfection, 135-138
Dispensing, 127-128
Dispensing Final Dosage Forms, 8
Disposable personal protective equipment, 40
Disposal, 143, 154
Documentation and Standard Operating Procedures, 9
Doffing, 35, 38, 114
   area, 98, 100
   order, 41-42
Donning, 35, 38
   order, 41-42
Double-gloving, 28, 43
Drug
   assay, 140
   classes, 24, 28
   returns, segregating, 67
   transport to infusion area, 39
Dual shoe covers, 47

E

Elastomeric half-mask, 36, 56
Elimination, 17
Emergency situations, 13, 116-117
Employee
   acknowledgment of risk by, 29
   consent form for, 34
   health issue and, 29
Enforceable standard, 1
Engineering controls, 17, 71
Entity, 3, 11, 15
Environmental monitoring, 139-141
Environmental Protection Agency (EPA), 3, 14, 76, 143
Environmental Quality and Control, 8
Environmental Services
   floor cleaning by, 135
   personnel of, 14
Estrogen, 56
Exhaust air, 96
Exposure types, 17-18
External shipping containers, 58
External venting, 74, 89
Eye contact, direct, 154, 166
Eye protection, 48, 154
Eye wash station, 152
Eyeglasses, 48

F

Face shield, 48
Facilities, 15
   design of, 82-93, 152
Facilities and Engineering Controls, 7
Feeding tube administration, 132
Final dosage form, 17-18, 20, 27
Finasteride, 21
Finished dosage form, 113, 125-126
   to ambulatory patients, 128
Finishes, 104-105
Fixed walls, 87

Flammable cabinet, 61, 64
Flexible wall surface, 87
Floor decontamination, 137
Fluconazole, 56
Fluorouracil, 140
    as cream, 27, 61
Food and Drug Administration (FDA), 14, 20, 33
    cleared devices, 84
Fosphenytoin, 116
    as infusion, 13

G

Gap analysis, 147
Genotoxins, 19
Germicidal agents, 136
Glossary, 9
Gloves, 42-44
    changing, 131
Good Distribution Practices, 12
Gown, 44-47, 164
    changing based on permeation information, 46
    impervious, 39
    permeability of, 44
Guideline, 12

H

Hair covers, 47
Hand hygiene, 35
Hand washing, 56, 116
Handling
    hazardous drugs, 13
    noninjectables, 162
Handling of Hazardous Drugs, 133
Hazard Communication Plan, 33
Hazard Communication Program, 8
Hazardous chemical, 33
Hazardous drug, 18, 151-152
    types of, 19
Hazardous waste, 14, 143
Hazmat, 146
HEPA filters, 72, 73
    redundant, 74
Home care HD pumps, 121
Home healthcare workers, 15
Hospital list, 19, 23-24

I

Ifosfamide, 140
IM methotrexate, 132
Injection storage, 60
International Standards Organization (ISO) 7, 63, 94, 97, 113, 153
    cleanroom, 5, 89
        positive pressure anteroom, 87
Introduction and Scope, 7
Inventory, 59
Investigational drugs, 21
Isolation gowns, 45
Isolator glove, 43

J

Joint Commission, 12

L

Labeling, 20, 112, 114
Labeling, Packaging, Transport, and Disposal, 8
Laminar air flow hood, 75, 77
Laminar air flow workbench, 77, 78
Lidded plastic storage bins, 68
Life cycle of hazardous drug, 13
List of Hazardous Drugs, 7
Literature, 12
Lot number records, 116
Low volume, 4, 90
    exemption, 103-104
Low-lint wipes, 115

M

Mail-order pharmacies, 11
Manipulation, 13, 24, 27, 124-125
Manual packaging, 27
Manual repackaging, 13
Manual unit-dose system, 123
Manufacturers, 15
Manufacturing personnel, 11-12
Medical Surveillance, 9

Medical Surveillance for Health Care Workers Exposed to Hazardous Drugs, 29, 30
Medical surveillance program, 29, 155
Megesterol, 20-21
  oral suspension, 27-28
Methotrexate, 55, 66, 140
  as tablets, 28, 61, 75, 112
  for ectopic pregnancy, 117
  in emergency room, 113
Microbial monitoring, 139
Misoprostol, 124
Mitomycin for ophthalmic use, 117
Modular cleanrooms, 87
Modular design, 96
Monoclonal antibodies (MABs), 20, 24
Mortar and pestle, disposable, 116
Must, use of, 4

N

N95 respirator, 38, 49, 50
Nasogastric tube tablet crushing, 125
National Institute for Occupation Safety and Health (NIOSH), 3, 12, 14, 29, 124, 143
  Alert on Preventing Occupational Exposure to Antineoplastic and Other Hazardous Drugs in Health Care Settings, 18
  Hierarchy of Controls, 17
  list, 3, 18-19, 28, 60, 74, 76, 78, 113, 128, 131, 147, 152-152
  list updates, 19
  performance protocol for CSTDs, 84
Negative buffer room door, 97
Negative pressure area, 56, 78-79, 88-89, 92
  HD opening in, 53
Negative pressure cabinet, 62, 64
Negative pressure cleanroom, 104
Negative pressure room, 4-5, 37-38, 59-60, 87, 90-91, 96-97
  access, 92
  inventory transport and, 66
  oral, injectable HDs and, 67
  range, 87
  requirements, 85
  storage in, 65-66
Negative pressure technique, 116, 118-119
New drug, 18-19, 32

Night nursing supervisors, 32
Non-antineoplastic drugs, 19, 24, 28, 42, 97
  oral solutions of, 112
  packaging of, 68
  storage of, 65
Nonsterile compounding, 39, 88, 152-153
  C-PEC and, 73-76
  PPE and, 42
Nonsterile hazardous drugs, 17
  non-antineoplastic compounding, 88
NSF Certified Biosafety Cabinetry, 72, 77
NSF/ANSI Standard 49, 80, 93
Nurses, 14
Nursing
  competencies, 133
  CSTD use and, 84
  station, 11
  unit storage area, 66
Nursing home, 11

O

Occasional nonsterile compounding, 74, 91
Occupational exposure limits, 33
Occupational risk, 12
Occupational Safety and Health Administration (OSHA), 3, 33, 152
  direct skin or eye contact and, 166
  Hazard Communication Standard, 33, 53
  respirator fit-testing and, 50
  Safety and Health Topics, 12
  training, 129
Occupational safety plan, 29, 37
OMB, 84
On-call pharmacist, 117
Oncology Nursing Society, 3, 29, 133
Oncology support medication, 64
Oral antineoplastic agents
  counting of, 69
  packaging of, 68
Oral hazardous drug, 61-62
  administration of, 131
Oral tablets, 123
Organotoxins, 19
Outpatient infusion, 133
Outpatient pharmacy, 15

Oxytocin
  drip, stat, 132
  pre-mixed, 133

P

Packaging hazardous drugs, 28, 36-37, 60, 68-70, 123-126
  large quantities and, 64
  of non-antineoplastics, reproductive hazards, 68
Packaging machine, 125
Parenteral administration, 131
Pass-through chamber, 92-93, 101-102
Pass-through refrigerator, 93, 101-102, 103
Pass-through window, 101
Patient carts, 129
Patient counseling, 38
Patient-specific antineoplastic doses, 124
Personal protective equipment (PPE), 8, 17, 153-154
  administration and, 131
  cleaning and, 135
  donning, doffing order for, 41
  eye protection and, 48
  generally, 35-42
  gloves and, 42-44
  gowns and, 44-47
  hair covers and, 47
  handling precautions and, 126
  receiving personnel and, 56
  respiratory protection and, 49-51
  reuse of, 40
  shoe covers and, 47
Personal Protective Equipment for Health Care Workers Who Work with Hazardous Drugs, 36, 37
Personnel, 14
  training of, 32
Personnel Training, 8
Pharmaceutical wholesalers, 12
Pharmacist checking, 37-38
  of formulation, 40
Pharmacy delivery drivers, 14
Phosphenytoin, 24
Physician practice nurses, 14
Plastic curtains, drapes, 87, 96
Plastic pouches, 132
Plastic-backed preparation mat, 114-115
Platinum-based agents, 140

Pneumatic tube, 66, 128, 129
Positive pressure area/room, 53, 84
Powder hood, 54, 71, 74-77, 94, 124
Powders, 17, 107
Predominant air, 91
Pre-filters, 74
Pregnant employee, 29-30
Pre-meds, 77
Pre-packaging, 123, 124
Pre-saturated gauze, 115
Pressure gauges, 89
Pre-sterilization areas for weighing powders, 94-95
Primary engineering control (PEC), 32, 88
  placement of, 85
Printer, 104
Protective gowns, 36

Q

Quality assurance, 139
Quality control, 139, 141

R

Raw material, 107
Ready-to-use dosage, 27-28, 125, 126
Receiving, 8, 56-57
  of hazardous drug shipments, 58
Receiving area, pressure monitoring, 55
Receiving personnel, 36
  elastomeric half-mask for, 50
  personal protective equipment for, 56, 58
  training of, 53-58
Redundant HEPA filters, 74-75
References, 10
Refrigeration, 63
Refrigerator, 104
  placement of, 65, 102-103
Regulations, 14
Reproductive capability, 33
Reproductive hazards, 19, 24, 97, 132
  packaging of, 68
  storage of, 65
Reproductive toxins, 19
Resource Conservation and Recovery Act (RCRA), 154-155

Respirator, 38, 49, 50, 154
Respiratory protection, 36, 38, 49-51
    fit-testing for, 50
Responsibilities of Personnel Handling Hazardous Drugs, 7
Reusable gown service, 46
Reusable mops, 138
Revisions, 1
Rituximab, 20
Robotic transport, 129
Roll-up door, 93
Rusty hood, 138

S

Safe Handling of Hazardous Drugs, 29, 30
Safety Data Sheet, 33, 145
Saline vials, 64
Scope, 4, 11
Segregated room, 79
Separate, 88
Shelving, 104
Shoe covers, 47
Should, use of, 4
Signage, 61
Single dose liquidation preparation, 75
Sinks, 104
    placement of, 92
Skin contact, direct, 154, 166
Small Entity Compliance Guide for Employers That Use Hazardous Chemicals, 33
Sodium thiosulfate, 136, 137
Solid final form, 33
Solid oral antineoplastics, 123
    packaging of, 68
Spill action plan, 147-148
Spill cleanup, 40, 146, 165-166
Spill Control, 9
Spill drill, 146, 147
Spill kit, 145-146, 165
Spills, 145-148, 154
    eye protection and, 48
    respiratory protection and, 51
Spray bottles, 115
Standard, 12
Sterile 70% isopropyl alcohol (sIPA), 43
Sterile chemotherapy gloves, 43, 44

Sterile compounding, 39, 153
    C-PEC, 76-81
Sterile hazardous drugs, 17
Storage, 59-67
    of investigational drugs, 21
Substitution, 17
Supplemental engineering control (SEC), 71, 72, 73
    cleaning, 88, 136
Supplier packaging, 58
Suppliers, 15
Supply chain personnel, 11-12
Surface
    finishes, 93
    sampling, 139, 140
Surgical masks, 49, 50

T

Tablet
    crushing, 18, 112, 124
    crushing by nurse, 131-132
    cutting, 5
    solutions, 18
    splitting, 112
Tackle box transport, 66
Technical Assistance Bulletin on Handling Cytotoxic Drugs in Hospitals, 3
Teratogenic drugs, 19, 20
Thiotepa, 44
Topical cream/drug, 21, 113
Totes
    delivery in, 55
    use of, 56
Transport, 36, 128, 129
Trash removal, 39
Types of Exposure, 7

U

Unclassified room/space, 89, 91
Un-gowning area, 98, 100
Uninterrupted power source ventilation, 105
Unit dosing, 123
Unit-dose methothrexate tablets, 75
Unit-dose package, 28, 68
    administration, 128

Unit-dosing, 28
    of liquids, 125
Unit-of-dose antineoplastic receipt, 55
Unit-of-use packages, 68
Unpacking, room, 54
USP <795>, 4, 11
    training, 32
    wording in, 13
USP <797>, 4, 11, 29, 33, 152
    facilities design, 85-86
    gown reuse, 45
    training, 32
    wording in, 13
USP Compounding Compendium
    hazardous drugs in, 1
    subscription to, 1
    updates for, 1

V

Valproic acid, 116
Vented to the outside, 89
Ventilation alarm, 81
Venting, 73-74, 76, 78
Vial, 20
Volatile agents/vapors, 62, 74
Volunteers, 129

W

Wall requirements, 87
Warfarin, 24, 56
    tablet cutting/splitting, 125
Washable gowns, 45
Waste hauler list, 20
Wholesaler, 15, 56
    tote opening, 54
Wipe sampling, 138, 140, 141
Wording, 13
Work gloves, 36
Work practices, 23, 36, 154-155